DON'T THINK

ABOUT MONKEYS

EXTRAORDINARY STORIES BY PEOPLE WITH TOURETTE SYNDROME

Edited By

Adam Ward Seligman

and

John S. Hilkevich

Don't Think About Monkeys
by *Adam Ward Seligman and John S. Hilkevich*

Published by: □┬○ **Hope Press** P.O.Box 188
Duarte, CA 91009-0188 U.S.A.
SAN 200-3244

Other books on Tourette syndrome by Hope Press:
Tourette Syndrome and Human Behavior
by *David E. Comings, M.D.*
Ryan – A Mother's Story of Her Hyperactive/Tourette Syndrome
Child by *Susan Hughes*
Hi, I'm Adam by *Adam Buehrens*
Adam and the Magic Marble by *Adam and Carol Buehrens*
Echolalia by *Adam Ward Seligman*
(to order see back leaf)

Library of Congress Cataloging-in-Publication Data

Don't think about monkeys : extraordinary stories by people with
Tourette syndrome / edited by Adam Ward Seligman and John S. Hilkevich.
    p.   cm.
  ISBN 1-878267-33-7 : $12.95
  1. Tourette syndrome - - Case studies.
I. Seligman, Adam Ward.1961- .   II. Hilkevich, John S., 1954 - .
RC375.D66 1992   92-15489
                                                        CIP

TABLE OF CONTENTS

Foreward   *Oliver Sacks*   i

Acknowledgements   *Adam Ward Seligman*   v
John S. Hilkevich

Introduction   *Adam Ward Seligman*   1
John S. Hilkevich

Doing it Differently   *Mitchell Vitiello*   9

Uncute, Unendearing   *Adam DePrince*   19

Subway People   *Frank Brancaccio*   29

In the Blink of an Eye   *Adam Ward Seligman*   33

In Walked Maura   *Maura Woodruff*   57

A Better Person   *Matt Foulkrod*   73

Just an Ordinary Kid   *Kevin R. Pratt*   79

Purpose   *Wayne Martin*   87

Three at a Time   *Rose Wood*   95

The Family Tourette   *Richard Stickann*   101

Cycles of Misery   *Marilyn Johnson*   121

Table of Contents

Making Friends with
   Tourette syndrome   *John S. Hilkevich*   133

Min Egen Lille Verden
   (My Own Little World) *Christian Melbye Jr.*   157

Rhythm Man   *David R. Aldridge*   173

In the Group: Life at
   a Tourette Syndrome
   Conference   *Adam Ward Seligman*   183

Afterthoughts   *John S. Hilkevich*
                         Adam Ward Seligman   195

Other Hope Press Books   201

FOREWORD

by

Oliver Sacks

We have many medical accounts of Tourette syndrome, but far too few stories "from the inside," stories of what it is like, what it means, to live with Tourette syndrome, every day and minute of one's life; how others respond to it, and how, finally, hopefully, one may come to terms with it. This collection of fifteen personal accounts gives a vivid sense of all the different ways in which Tourette syndrome may affect a person – for it is never the same in any two people – of the sufferings and complex social difficulties it may cause, but equally of the great

---

Dr. Sacks is author of the enormously successful books, The Man Who Mistook His Wife for a Hat and Awakenings. The latter formed the basis of an equally successful movie.

range of resources (human and social, no less than medical) which can turn a tormented or disabled life into a decent, even creative, one.

Some of the narratives in *Don't Think about Monkeys* are from young children or adolescents – the first generation, as the editors point out, to get a prompt diagnosis of Tourette syndrome.

Other accounts relate what used to be all but universal – a delay of ten or twenty or more years, years of deep uncertainty, and sometimes accusations, before the diagnosis was made. One sees how the diagnosis itself is sometimes ambiguous: it ends the uncertainty, the misapprehensions, but it carries the implication of a lifelong disorder.

Some of the pieces in this collection are deeply harrowing, even shocking, such as the finely written *In Walked Maura,* by Maura Woodruff, where the intensity of Tourette, and its power of alienation, moves a young woman to thoughts of desperation and death, though (finally) to poetry, and liberating creativity.

There are painful accounts of complex family difficulties, teasing at school, discrimination by employers, rejection or stigmatization by neighbors and others. But what comes through, finally, is something very positive – that with increasing education about, and awareness of, Tourette syndrome, life for those with Tourette is improving, and that the incomprehending and often cruel attitudes of the past are tending to give way now to increased acceptance and understanding. This important change is something which would not have occurred without the unremitting efforts of Touretters themselves, and of their organization, the Tourette Syndrome Association.

But it is not just "coping" or "accepting" – rather bland states – which come through in these accounts, but sometimes something much more. I felt this especially in *Rhythm Man*, a marvelous account of a Tourettic musician, and how his Tourette and his musicianship can fuse:"Rhythm and Tourette syndrome have been intertwined," David Aldridge writes, "from the first day I found that drumming on a table could mask my jerky hand, leg and neck movement . . . could harness my unbounding [Tourettic] energy, directing it into an orderly flow." Aldridge describes how, with jazz, the "rollercoaster ride" of Tourette could be transformed, because he was riding it, controlling it, not it him. This, for him, is the other side of Tourette – Tourette as, potentially, a gift of energy, not a curse.

Another favorite piece of mine in this book is the final one, by Adam Ward Seligman, *In the Group*, because this goes beyond the situation of the individual Touretter who lives alone, isolated, with his Tourette, and considers the community he may participate in and enjoy. Here Seligman describes the three great meetings (Cincinnati 1987, McLean 1989 and 1991) which brought together young adults with Tourette from all over the country, and indeed all over the world, and showed them the possibility of a sort of Tourette brotherhood or community. "It was here," he writes, "that my search for community ended." And, at another one of the great get-togethers, "These were the dearest people of my life and I had only known most of them for three days." Seligman speaks in the warmest terms of "a Tourette community," and of how, with half a dozen others, he formed such a community, for three days, in the Ozarks.

Even though such intimacy, such community, is of necessity rare, one can learn to be on good, and even friendly, terms with one's Tourette – this is the central theme of John Hilkevich's remarkable piece, *Making Friends with Tourette Syndrome*, in which he speaks of the pluses and minuses, the transparency, the intensity, of Tourette (at least, so far as he himself has experienced it):

"Tourette syndrome is integrated into my spirituality. It has been both a curse and a gift. It has both isolated and connected me. . . With the [same] intensity of a Tourettic tension, I can feel in my body the hop of a rabbit or the surrender of a hawk in flight to the winds. I physically and emotionally feel the life force gushing from the wound of an injured animal or leaking from a plucked tomato . . . How thin and transparent are the boundaries of life and death!"

Some people with Tourette syndrome may be maintained on medication, with such control of their Tourette that they can all but forget it. But for those who cannot be pharmacologically "controlled" – or who, perhaps, as adults, may decide they do not wish to be – there is, finally, beyond mere "coping" or "acceptance," this possibility of a profound integration as Hilkevich describes; and this, perhaps, is the deepest theme of a fascinatingly varied book.

ACKNOWLEDGMENTS

Many people gave generously of their time in making this book a reality. First and most important is Mary Lou Reaver, Executive Director of the Pennsylvania Tourette Syndrome Association, who introduced me to John S. Hilkevich and led Frank Branccaccio to us. I also want to thank my dear friend Pete Olson for telling me the parable that became our title.

Among the people who read the text, and made comments, I would like to thank my sister Lucy Kanazawa for her editorial skills, and her patience with what became a deluge of faxes – her prompt attention was a godsend; my brother Brad Seligman; my mother Muriel; Neva Duyndam of Duvall Media, Inc. for the editing of *In The Blink of an Eye*; my friend Lynn Sagramoso for her comments on the text and the back cover photograph; my friend Mary Kennedy, President of the Metropolitan Detroit Tourette Syndrome association for both her insights and her daughter, Elisabeth Archambault, who taught me so much about friendship and trust; my publicists Bobbi Marcus and Lori

Hehr for helping with the *Echolalia* tour and promotion on this book; warm thanks to Oliver Sacks for his support of Tourette writers everywhere; and most of all thanks to our publisher David Comings M.D. for his vision of Hope Press and believing in this project.

Adam Ward Seligman

Within two days after mailing my first autobiographical account of my Tourette syndrome experience to the National Tourette Syndrome Association, Sue Levi called me, resulting in a conversation full of bubbling-over support and encouragement. Further validation of my stepping-out came from Mary Lou Reaver of the Pennsylvania Tourette Syndrome Association and from the many people of the Tourette Syndrome Association community who wrote and called me during that amazing and hectic month. To them, and Debbie Clark, Kim Greene, their families in our local Tourette Syndrome Chapter chapter, and to Bob Nast to whom I owe far more than I can list here, I can heartfully declare, I love you and thank you.

Overall, I dedicate my portion of this book, my portion of its energy to those loved ones in the sidelines, who never abandoned me, including the several friends mentioned in my chapter, and equally important one's who were not; but mainly to my parents, John and Marcella, and my sister, Evelyn, the three humans on this earth who have never ceased to hold the loving and reflective and unconditional acceptance of God's love and face, as I grew up and out. I am grateful to them and to the incarnation of son Jason, who obviously manifests a promise to be a teacher to all of us.

John S. Hilkevich

INTRODUCTION

There is a story about an Indian businessman who heard about a holy man who could walk on water. The businessman reasoned that if he could walk on water the publicity would help his business. He decided to seek out the holy man.

The holy man heard the businessman's interest in walking on water and agreed to take him as a disciple. "All you need to do is follow these meditations, stop eating these foods and read these prayers. Then you can walk on water like me."

The businessman smiled with delight. "That is it? Wonderful. I'll start today." He headed for the door.

The holy man cleared his throat. "There is just one more thing. It's a little thing but very important."

The businessman stood in the doorway impatiently. "Yes?"

"Don't think about monkeys."

Introduction

Inside the businessman's head a stream of monkeys appeared; waltzing, dancing, eating and playing. He walked out the door and saw two monkeys by his car. As he drove home he pictured every monkey he had ever seen in a book. That night monkeys swung through his dreams. Within a week he was monkey mad.

Having Tourette syndrome is a lot like not thinking about monkeys. The monkeys are the tics, vocalizations, urges, obsessions, behaviors and enactments that are with us constantly, overwhelming our daily lives. To live and function we have to keep the Tourette syndrome at bay – we have to try not to think about monkeys. This book is about how fourteen people with Tourette syndrome survive and grow in their lives despite all those damn monkeys.

But before you read these stories of peoples lives you need to understand what Tourette syndrome is. Since it was first described accurately over a hundred years ago by Dr. Georges Gilles de la Tourette, the misconceptions about this neurobehavioral disorder have challenged the lives of both those with it and those who treat it.

The popular conception of Tourette syndrome is of a movement disorder: tics. The second image is of the disease that makes people swear. The third image is that it is very rare and very severe. These are all true to a degree: people with the disorder must have a tic component to be correctly diagnosed; coprolalia (involuntary swearing) is present in about thirty percent of the people who have it; the full scale case is thankfully rare. But if that were all Tourette syndrome was, then this book wouldn't be needed.

Tourette syndrome is considered a very common genetic behavioral disorder characterized by a lack of inhibition. The inhibition may be around movement resulting in tics or twitches. It may be a problem inhibiting speech or

2

sound resulting in vocalizations. It may be a breakdown in thought or action resulting in obsessive compulsive disorder. In may be a breakdown in controlling one's concentration resulting in attention deficit disorder. It may even be a problem controlling emotion, like in the depression Maura writes about or the anger my grandfather was unable to suppress.

The most common form of Tourette syndrome is a problem of impulsivity: of controlling addictive behaviors. You'll read a lot about alcoholism in this book – it can be a part of the disease. It is also part of the solution as the tools people with substance abuse issues use – the twelve steps – are applied by John to Tourette syndrome in this book's conclusion.

Every aspect of behavior can be affected by Tourette syndrome. Yet the person with Tourette syndrome is not a loaded cannon waiting to explode. The miracle of tic suppression, or substitution, allows one to put off symptoms until a safe or appropriate place for them is found. For me it is my home. For others it is in the car, playing a musical instrument, or on the ball playing field. This hidden blessing of suppression, so painfully learned, so hard to develop, allows people with Tourette syndrome to find the accommodations in their lives that make it worth living. It is our way of not thinking about monkeys.

So enter what Christian calls "Our Tourette world." Linger awhile with people who seem very different from the average person you may know. And look in the mirror of the Tourette syndrome experience: You may see yourself looking back!

Adam Ward Seligman

Introduction

It was 7 AM in rural New York state. Sitting on a sofa in a group home for teenagers, sipping some coffee, I was nudged by a social worker.

"Watch this kid, Joe, he's the one," she whispered. A fifteen year old boy had just entered the living room area, stopping at the bottom of the stairs to bang his right foot three times on the floor before bringing his left down. He then turned to the wall, tapping that three times, spun around and walked into the room, tapping every piece of furniture as he went. My friend called him over and introduced us, upon which Joe sat abruptly next to me, tapping my leg and arm repeatedly. Within two minutes of small talk, he was telling me that he was in the program because his parents could not stand him. He made the same grunting noises I make while he spoke. I could see his stomach convulsing.

During the third minute of our conversation another teenager walked up and fulfilled his obligation to inform me how crazy and retarded Joe was, citing as evidence how "He touches people all the time, hits the walls, rocks in his chair, makes noises and other weird things." The good-intentioned helper warned me, "Be careful! He's strange!" I politely thanked him and assured him I knew how to handle people like Joe.

Joe, tapping me again while sniffing my shoulder, asked me, "I'm not retarded am I?" I looked right into his eyes, "Absolutely not. I do much of what you do, but I hide it better." His eyes widened, "You mean I'm not the only one?" While my heart hurt, we were interrupted before I could answer. Meanwhile, my social worker friend whispered again, "Do you think he has Tourette syndrome?" My eyes rocketed toward the ceiling and rolled back down. "Do I *think*? Joe has Tourette syndrome up the wazoo!" Now

4

there was a four minute diagnosis that would raise many a therapist's eyebrows.

Joe returned to my side and made me his friend, a friendship animated by his profound hunger for knowledge – about his pain, confusion, weird behavior, and inner demons. During my visit he shadowed me and that was the first day after seven months he volunteered to read aloud in his first class.

Why was I the first person he perceived as a resource of healing and hope? And why am I telling you about Joe? Because I have been through this scenario often with many boys and girls, men and women, like Joe. If they had epilepsy, cancer or diabetes, they would not need to do it alone or without the precious understanding needed. Nor would they be subjected to deteriorating self-fantasies. Joe did not need to be subjected to that either, but he was not understood by his parents, by his teachers, and, most shamefully of all, by his mental health workers.

Adam writes about his hunch that our generation may be the last that will be crushingly victimized by misdiagnosis and mistreatment. I hope so, but I am not so sure. We did make the kickoff and the younger generation will receive, but it seems it will be their children who must catch the pass and run to the goal. It is my hunch that Tourette syndrome will soon be recognized as one of the most common genetic disorders and behavioral drives. Sadly and ironically, I could see some of it in the same kids who were teasing Joe.

Muscular dystrophy was never described or reported until the middle of the nineteenth century. Within a couple of years of that, a prominent Parisian neurologist who taught Doctors Tourette and Freud, was struck enough by this to remark, "How come that a disease so common, so widespread, and so recognizable at a glance, is only recog-

nized now? Why did we need Duchenne to open our eyes?"
Twenty years after Duchenne, Gilles de la Tourette described another unrecognized syndrome. Charcot can now
ask, "Who will open our eyes to this?" The answer is
certainly not the mental health community, but from the
Tourette syndrome persons themselves, out of whose experience this book has grown.

When Adam first mentioned his intent to produce an
anthology, I told him he was reading my mind, from three
thousand miles away. Our visions harmonized and in
fifteen minutes Adam said, "Why don't we co-author the
book?" It was a leap of faith – a step beyond the edge – to
believe in and put energy into publishing a collection of
Tourette syndrome experiences from all over the country
and even overseas, to do it with someone I had never met
and will see only a couple of times before publication date,
someone who lives on the opposite coast, with a very
different personal history, upbringing and life-style. Adam
intrigued me with his personal comfortablility, acute wit,
perceptive observations and writing talent. I first felt honored then quickly felt humbled as the contributors of this
book made it transcend both of us. We were meant to be only
the channels of many voices – voices that welled up from
deep within the human psyche in which resides struggle and
desperation in the midst of misunderstanding, mislabeling
and outright abuse.

Neither Adam or I knew what would appear from our
uniting energies; our only parameters were to express the
diversity of Tourette syndrome and connect to the hearts of
all readers, not just those in the Tourette syndrome community. We were both surprised at the ultimate character the
book exuded. Considering the early literature on Tourette
syndrome and anecdotal documentation, there was a good

chance of the book reflecting the pessimism and sense of futility that comes with staring down a disease that is so far incurable, and all-intrusive into every facet of the persona; from walking, breathing, and learning, to sexuality and spirituality. Instead, you will read about journeys in healing, self-exploration, integration, and triumph. Interestingly enough, (you figure out why,) many of our contributors told us that while they would not want others to inherit the syndrome, they would be reluctant to give it up themselves. Let me just suggest that this points to the gift flip-side of any curse and the healing power of reframing bad pictures.

I finish by offering a sort of disclaimer for my Tourette syndrome friends: if an associate counselor invited me to interview someone who was suffering from "acute clinical depression" or from "anorexia," I could walk into the office predictably knowing what to expect and what I would witness. But if he or she asked me to see a person suffering from Tourette syndrome, I, a counselor, teacher, researcher and Tourette syndrome person myself, would still not know what to expect, as its symptoms are so diverse, so integrated into the personality, so complex, so multifaceted.

The point I'm making is that Adam does Tourette syndrome things I don't and vice versa. If you were in the same room with Adam, me, Maura, Kevin, Christian, and any other of our writers, you would decide we were all unique with our own idiosyncrasies and eccentricities . . . except, of course, if you were a paradigm-stuck therapist, in which case you would have a separate diagnosis for each of our obvious problems.

The bottom line message is to caution you against figuring all of us out based on our individual descriptions of our Tourette syndrome lives. We don't all vacuum our houses everyday, wash our hands every hour, touch each

Introduction

other as we talk, jump around or bang things, refuse to wear socks or underwear, wet our beds, have weekly nightmares, blink our eyes or bark like dogs, stare people into the uncomfort zone, drink alcohol, or count floor tiles, or reread every sentence three times. We do what we told you we do in this anthology.

Julius Caesar asked the Roman senate, "Lend me your ears." Please do just that, without the Roman follow-through. (They stabbed him.) I welcome, on behalf of the Tourette syndrome community, the lending of your ears and of your hearts. Such connections give birth to new life.

John S. Hilkevich

DOING IT DIFFERENTLY

by

Mitchell M. Vitiello

In "Afterthoughts," the final chapter of this book, I mention the explosion of letters I received after circulating, my first description of my Tourette syndrome experience and quoted from one. Here is another: "I have read your account of Tourette syndrome and have been greatly touched, for I believe I have some inkling of what this has been like. When I was a young teenager, I was troubled by some nervous condition that caused me to do things I abhorred . . . clacking rhythms with my teeth, flapping my elbows to my side, tapping my feet, etc. It was not involuntary, so perhaps it was not Tourette syndrome. But it was definitely compulsive and I had to hide myself away at times so I could "do it right" according to the rhythm my brain wanted to tap. It lasted some three years, probably linked to stress in junior and senior high school. Thank God I out grew it. I shuddered even to be reminded of this unhappy time in my life . . ."

Mitchell M. Vitiello

Just recently I interviewed a family whose son was just diagnosed with Tourette syndrome. Like the person I quoted above, the father "outgrew" Tourette syndrome and expressed two striking realizations: 1. What was ailing him as a youth was Tourette syndrome; and 2. He never connected his son's "habits" with his own experience.

Mitchell is another person who "outgrew" Tourette syndrome, the only one of our writers. He was told that "a small percentage grow out of it," but I wonder if that percentage would be much greater were it not for those who dismissed their childhood "nervous habits" as a parenthetic "stage" of growing up. Notably, Mitchell has not dismissed his Tourette syndrome experience but rather held onto what made him feel like "I'm going to die" as a source of strength and empowerment for his sensitive and compassionate spirit.

As a fourteen year old, Mitchell published his Tourette syndrome story in _Shoetree Magazine_ and in _Childlife_, as it appears here, ending with his letter to his father, and winning the National Association for Young Writers competition. Impressed by his article, I sought permission to use it in this book and asked Mitch to add an update. Now finishing high school, he reports how his symptoms may have dismissed him, but he has not dismissed them. They have shaped his plans to be " . . . an elementary school teacher. I want to start fresh and teach these children the right way of life, how to be sensitive, educated, polite. I want to help each of them to be able to stand alone as an individual." The highest validation I can give to a person is to welcome him or her to be a teacher to my son. You have my welcome, Mitch.

John S. Hilkevich

When I was eight, I noticed that I was different from the other kids. I made strange movements. It got to the point where the other kids noticed. They started to laugh and looked at me strangely. I felt bad inside and sometimes I cried. I didn't know what was wrong with me. My parents didn't know. The doctors didn't know either.

When I was in an airport waiting for a plane, I couldn't sit still in my chair. I would start to jerk violently, all over. There would be people trying to look like they weren't paying attention, but I could see that they were. My arms and legs would throw themselves toward the wall. My head would nod repeatedly. Eventually I would get a migraine headache from moving my head so much. I felt like leaving the airport and running away.

Sometimes when I would be walking home from school, I would notice that my shoulder would fly up and hit my ear or my feet would get this urge to kick. In class my head would jerk. I would try to control these movements but they would overrule me. It was like an incredible urge for them to get free and make me wiggle and jolt. There were times when it would go absolutely nuts. I would try to stay in the house and not go out to play for days. I was thinking, "I'm going to die," when it got really bad.

Reading and writing were always a problem for me. I could never keep a pencil still or read without my head jerking and losing my place. My homework was always taking me longer than it should.

It was better at home because my family was trying to help. They didn't know what it was so they called my movements "Mitch's habit." They didn't pay attention to it much and that was good for me because at home I could forget a little bit.

The years went by. I was nine, then ten, then eleven. All those years I developed new movements. Finally, when I was twelve, I was taken to special doctors who put things on my head, things that dug in and hurt, and I had tests and needles. The whole

11

thing. Then they figured it out. I have Tourette syndrome, a movement disorder that doctors think is caused by too much dopamine in the brain. It causes muscle movements, tics, and vocal sounds that cannot be controlled. They think it is caused by a problem with the neurotransmitters in the brain that carry signals from cell to cell along the nerves. There are medicines to control severe cases, but they have bad side effects. You can leave it alone and deal with the condition and problems such as people making fun of you. People with Tourette syndrome can expect to live a normal life span. Even though the tics can make a person look like he is nervous, it is not a nervous condition. Some lucky people grow out of it completely after adolescence. I was told I have a mild case.

The time I learned to deal with my problem was the summer I went to camp in Boston. It was 1987 and I was twelve and a half. I had looked forward all the months before going and the Tourette seemed not to be acting up. Suddenly, just before leaving for camp, I had an allergy attack that always seemed to start the Tourette's problem up. I was angry because I knew people would make fun of me at camp just like they did at school. It was frightening.

On the first day of camp, no one would even talk to me. I called home and told my parents that I had no friends. I was down and lonely. My mother wanted to come to pick me up. She thought the Tourette syndrome was the worst it ever had been. It was. But, my father said he had something very important to tell me. He said that I had to learn to deal with the condition, no matter how bad it got.

"If you act like it bothers you, it will bother other people. How you deal with your problem is how other people will deal with it. Act like it is nothing and soon they will forget about it."

That was my father's advice. I thanked him and hung up. I went up to my dorm to think about the advice he had given me.

The only choices I had were to go home, to stay and be miserable, or to take my father's advice.

All of the other times when people would make fun of me, or stare at me, I would feel sad inside, like a freak. I felt fed up with the whole situation and all the years I had been putting up with it. But it was still hard to break away from my old way of dealing with it.

I decided to take my father's advice. I thought about it all night and I figured I had nothing to lose. My heart was in it. I went for it the next morning.

At breakfast I sat at an empty table with my tray in front of me. My movements seemed worse than ever. My head kept on jerking back as I was trying to sip orange juice. Eating my eggs was a problem. My fork kept flying out of my hand.

As I kept eating, I saw five kids coming over to the table and I knew it was time for me to try my new technique. My first thing was to act differently than I ever did before. I didn't move away from the table and I didn't look down and try to pretend was invisible. My thoughts were positive. I kept on telling myself, "I am powerful. I will not let this bother me."

As the other kids sat, they noticed me right away. I saw them look at me and mumble to each other. I introduced myself. I said, "Hi, I'm Mitchell Vitiello. I'm from New Jersey. Where are you from?"

Two of the boys told me their names and where they were from. The other three just said "Hi." Already I knew it was starting to work. I was acting differently than I used to and they were responding differently than other kids had. A boy named Seth asked me why I was moving like that. I said to myself, "I must be strong. I must act like it doesn't bother me."

"Oh, it's just a condition that I have that acts up sometimes and makes me move differently. It's nothing major. It comes and goes. I can't help it. You'll get used to it," I said and smiled.

All the other kids went on eating and talking. I was over-whelmed at the outcome. I felt like letting out a big sigh of relief. I never felt that way in all the years that I had the condition. Here I had acted as if it didn't matter and the other kids didn't care either. My father's advice was good. I never expected it to work.

I learned a lot that summer. I felt good inside. Everywhere I went I used my new technique. It helped me tremendously. There were times when I was down, but not as down as I was before. Now, I had courage to go out and do whatever I wanted to do in confidence that I could achieve it.

I changed the way I used to react and people reacted in a different way to me. I have continued to use my father's advice and things have been a lot easier.

Last Father 's day I showed my gratitude to my father who gave me the advice that changed my life. This is the letter I sent him:

June 18, 1988

Dear Dad:

Happy Father's Day. I'd like to say that you're the greatest Dad a kid like me could ever have. Why? Because you're always there when I need an arm to rest on and to cry when I'm feeling down. But the greatest thing about you is that you teach me right from wrong. I am growing up now and learning new things and experiences that I never knew before. Without your support and kindness I would never have made it to where I am today. I have a sense of direction and best of all a caring father. I love you Dad. I am proud to be your son.

Love,
Mitch

After camp, I entered eighth grade. The Tourette syndrome symptoms were similar to how they were in camp. I was asked by many kids what was wrong. I told them it was a syndrome called Tourette and I proceeded to tell them about the symptoms. Some of them were immature and laughed at me which made me feel different and others would tease me behind my back and I would hear about it later. Those were the kind of days when the bathroom was my only friend. I always picked the place in the corner of the bathroom where the mirrors and non-see-through windows were. It was a good place to let out anger and sadness. No one would ever see me because it was away from the entrance to the bathroom. Someday I would spend half an hour just pitying myself for no other reason than Tourette. I would constantly be having to wipe my face from the tears that kept dripping from my eyes. After that, I would feel good enough to go back to class.

An amazing thing happened that year which really surprised me. Although some of the kids hurt me in many ways, there were some I told about Tourette syndrome who totally understood. Some of them even wanted to hear more about it. After that, I knew my father's advice really works in all situations and not just as it did at camp. That made me feel great. That year, I finally came to grips with what I had and started to face people head on.

The next year, ninth grade, a miraculous thing happened. I did not notice it right away. Everyday I would come to school and go to classes like I always did. I found that my Tourette syndrome wasn't as active as always. It cooled down. It got to the point when I would have tics and make noises only 10, maybe 15, times a day. Then, after a while, it was less. I was only having tics occasionally. Toward the end of the year, I stopped being asked questions such as "What is that you're doing?" or "What's with you, pal?"

I felt normal for once in my life. I could walk down those halls just like anybody else I knew. By the end of the year, the

15

miracle happened. My Tourette syndrome symptoms seemed completely gone. Very rarely did I ever jerk anymore. I was so happy. My mom told me that statistics show only a small percentage of kids with Tourette syndrome completely grow out of it and I seemed to be in that group.

By the end of that year, I got a job at a nursing home as a volunteer to run bingo. It seemed like the perfect job to do. I would get a chance to help someone else. Things in my own life were so much better.

For two years I worked at the Oak Ridge Manor Nursing Home. I would come every Sunday and set up and announce the numbers for bingo.

It was so satisfying to see those old, old people look up to me as a father figure. If I called a number and someone wouldn't hear me, they would ask me to help them. Some seniors did not know how to play the game and they would want me to play with them by their table. When I would go over to help the senior, the others would want me at their table to help them. Some of them were senile and told me to tell them what they were doing repeatedly.

It was sometimes lots of fun and there were good jokes being shared. After the game was over, everybody was thankful. Some kissed and hugged me and kept saying, "Oh, he is so dear to give up his Sundays to play with us. There are a lot of things he could have been doing." I didn't mind at all helping the seniors and I didn't consider it a waste of a Sunday at all.

Every Sunday, after bingo, I would go visit these two quadriplegic men on the second floor. These men couldn't wait for me to come each week because when I came I was able to help them by changing the station on their television set and read them their cards and mail. These men were totally unable to speak, move, walk. They lie in hospital beds all day and night until they eventually will pass away.

One of the men, Stanley, is a very nice man. We communicated by him mouthing out words. He gets tired very easily so, if I didn't get what he was trying to say the first time, I wouldn't get it repeated. I felt that it was similar to having Tourette syndrome because when I would try to explain, it was hard to make people understand. Only I knew what I was trying to express.

Stanley and I had many things in common. He gets really lonely. He can't move all day. He rarely gets any visitors. Just like me when I had the symptoms of Tourette syndrome.

I spent most of my time with Stanley when I was there, because Doug, the other fellow, did not want to be bothered with me trying to make him cheerful. I could really understand where he was coming from. I used to be like Doug, not wanting people to notice me. I felt lost and lonely and if I tried to cheer up, I'd still be depressed. I guess that is how Doug felt.

The things I did for the nursing home really made me feel good about myself. It made me feel like I just did not take, but I gave something back. What I gave back wasn't close to what I got from the experience I gained in that nursing home.

In 10th grade, I was still in Barnstable Academy, a private school, for half the year. Then, I transferred to public high school in my own town. It had a lot more people. In the other school, there was only a total of 100 to 150 students, if that, and I wanted to be with more people. I was really high-spirited about myself when I made that move.

During the rest of that school year, it took me a while to get used to the facilities in the new school that my old one didn't have. It took me almost all of the rest of the year to get adjusted.

As of today, 1991, I am living a normal life without any symptoms of Tourette syndrome. Occasionally, food allergies, which seem in my case to stir up a few symptoms, give me a problem, but not often. I am in my junior year of high school. I plan to graduate and go on to college to study to be an elementary school teacher. I want to start fresh and teach these children the right way of life, how to be sensitive, educated, polite. I want to help each of them to be able to stand alone as an individual.

Perhaps, that was the hardest thing for me to learn.

TOURETTE SYNDROME: UNCUTE, UNENDEARING

by

Adam DePrince

Adam DePrince is so Tourettic that he cannot use a pen to write out checks or sign his name to documents. His muscular tics were timed at 200 a minute. They caused a painful swelling of the neck from an unrelenting build up of lactic acid. Before entering school his parents were told he would be institutionalized. Later, in junior high school, he was informed he would not "amount to anything." Sometimes one cannot even hold a phone conversation with Adam. The phone flies out of his hands or his head keeps jerking him away from the transmitter making a simple conversation an impossibility. One wonders, "Who is this guy I am trying to talk to? He can't even sign his name to a letter, which are always done on his computer."

The guy we talked to has been appointed to the Mayor's

Adam DePrince

Advisory Council (for handicapped persons) in Cherry Hill, New Jersey. He is the co-editor of a Micro-computer users newsletter for the New Jersey Institute of Technology. He is an 'A' average Computer Science college freshman who tested out of so many courses he expects to achieve his Master's degree four years from this writing and a first year college student with the distinction of being assigned independent research by his mathematics professor. He is constantly sought by juniors and seniors for his tutelage.

According to the present educational paradigm, a person who cannot write out a check at age eighteen is learning disabled. (Interestingly enough, up to half of all Tourette syndrome persons are classified as learning disabled.) But Adam could not write due to his muscular tics. He would be so slow at arithmetic computations because, before producing the final answer, he had to check it obsessively through three mathematical base systems so he could trust his final calculation. Child study evaluators would judge him as slow and disabled by their criteria. Given a turning of the tables, they could never meet his criteria for arriving at a final computation. Adam has and will continue to outperform his instructors. His performance is a message, reinforced by many others I have interviewed, to evaluators that Tourette syndrome and Obsessive Compulsive Disorder can render the appearance of a learning disability, while, in reality, they are looking at a convoluted expression of genius.

Adam's juxtaposition of perceptions of various handicaps prompted us to use his story as a set-up for the context of our other writer's contributions. It is an endearing story of an unendearing disorder.

John S. Hilkevich

Tourette syndrome: Uncute, Unendearing

Danny, a preschooler with Spina Bifida, scoots about in his candy apple red wheelchair, engaging everyone in conversations about football, or tractor trailers. It takes the personality of an ogre to be able to ignore Danny. Most people, including strangers, crouch down to chat with him. There is something about a kid in a wheelchair that brings out the best in everyone.

Five year old Nancy is petite and flirtatious. She is also deaf. This combination of features just tugs at your heartstrings. At least it did to mine, for when I took Nancy's older sister, Lindsey, to my high school Junior prom I brought flowers for both Lindsey and Nancy. I'm not the only sucker in town. When Nancy bats those long black lashes and lets out a squeal of glee, no one can resist her.

Adam, with his large sky-blue eyes, rosy cheeks, and curly hair should be an irresistible two and a half year old. When the sweet, elderly woman in the supermarket pats him on the head, and tries to engage his attention, he lets out a bloodcurdling shriek. He nearly throws himself out of the shopping cart. This kindly senior citizen has just interrupted his tally of grocery products that begin with the letter "B." He needed to remember them in the exact order in which his shopping cart passed them. He is now in aisle thirteen! He screams, inconsolable, because he knows that his mother will not walk up and down each and every aisle letting him recheck his list.

Adam's mother isn't necessarily unreasonable. She just can't figure out why her child is screaming, because Adam still can't talk. What his mother doesn't yet know is that her son has been reading since he was a little more than a year old. There is a method to his madness that she can't even imagine. She is embarrassed and confused. The unsuspecting elderly woman no longer finds him at all appealing. Muttering, she moves as far away as possible to avoid him.

Adam is three and a half years old. It is the Sunday of the "Family Picnic." He has spent most of the day crying. He still can't talk. His aunts and uncles are having a tough time showing affection for him. His grandparents are clearly frustrated. He needs to count to five hundred backwards and forwards in his head without pause. Every time somebody comes over to hug or kiss him he loses his place. He'll never finish doing this perfectly. He'll never get it just right. He can't enjoy himself until he does this just right, but everyone keeps bothering him. He is in a frenzy of frustration and anxiety.

Adam has been diagnosed by physicians at two major medical centers as having Infantile Autism. They point the finger of blame at his mother. After all, this is 1976, and the words of Bruno Bettleheim's Empty Fortress ring in their minds. His parents have been told that he probably will be institutionalized before he is five years old.

Adam is not autistic. Many years pass before Adam is correctly diagnosed as having full blown Tourette syndrome. Besides the motor and vocal tics (and later coprolalia) Adam always had a really red-hot case of Obsessive-Compulsive Disorder.

It was the Obsessive-Compulsive Disorder that caused Adam to work all of his math problems in binary, then base sixteen, before he could work them in the standard decimal system. It was the time consuming rituals of OCD that made him perpetually late for the school bus. It was the mind rituals of counting, reciting and categorizing that made it difficult to get words out of his mouth. While struggling to speak with his peers he would flap his arms, rub his chest and roll his eyes.

In the eyes of his elementary and junior high school teachers, he was stubborn and resistant to their suggestions, or . . . daydreaming. Daymaring was probably more like it, as he chased math problems through three base systems.

The Dannys and Nancys of the world are always thought to be cute and endearing. The Adams of the world, victims of Tourette syndrome, are not. The Dannys and Nancys of the world are perceived as handicapped. The Adams are usually perceived at best as "very strange." I should know. I'm Adam.

What I am sharing is not a whine of self pity. I was most fortunate in having parents who, although confused by my behavior, were nonetheless convinced that it was some type of physical disability that needed to be understood. They were always realistic in their expectations. They always shared their ideas, as well as medical findings with me. They convinced me at an early age that I was not "weird." I had a medical problem. Now I recognized how courageous they were to take a stand that flew in the face of conventional medicine. They fought many battles for my cause.

My parents' efforts to understand my "odd" behaviors, while also praising and encouraging my talents, helped me to develop an unusually strong sense of self-confidence. My mother spent years searching for a medical answer that would vindicate our belief in my psychological stability. She found the answer for me with the diagnosis of Tourette syndrome.

Armed with correct information of my "medical" diagnosis of the neurological disorder, Tourette syndrome, I am often, but not always, able to change first impressions. This has been helpful when dealing with open minded professionals, close friends and kind acquaintances. Unfortunately, it doesn't help a lot when dealing with close-minded professionals, and acquaintances who would rather laugh and ridicule, than learn and accept.

When I went off to college I was full of self-confidence and enthusiasm. I had a S.A.T. score of 1450. I had graduated from high school with honors. I had been elected to the Senior Hall of Fame. Thanks to the help of my high school's staff and administrators I had experienced harassment only once, briefly, in my Sophomore year. Only three high school teachers, out of many, thought that I was somehow inferior. I had an outstanding guidance counselor whose understanding of me as a person, and Tourette syndrome as a disorder, helped me over rough spots. I had friends, dates and proms to remember. The negative experiences of my early childhood had long since been filed away.

My high school was Camelot. I'm in the real world now and though I am finding that more people are becoming aware of Tourette syndrome, and the difficulties of its victims, even today, in spite of the media attention given to this disorder, the empathy that is given to the wheelchair user, deaf, blind, and amputee, is often denied to victims of Tourette syndrome.

My first semester of college was extraordinarily educational. Most of my learning occurred outside the classroom. Although I was attending a highly competitive university in New England, close to centers for Tourette syndrome research, ignorance was rife.

I made a few close friends in this college, but nothing could compensate for the harassment and suffering that I experienced in my dorm. Education is the key to understanding, but when the administration fails to educate, then how do you deal with a drunken student who thinks that it's open season on the weird kid down the hall? How can the administration educate if the dean assigned to disabled students states, "Well, Adam isn't really handicapped. We have two kids in wheel chairs in our school."

Is it a handicap to be unable to walk down the hall to the bathroom, because your tics have been so exacerbated by the students across the hall who have set a pea shooter in their peek hole, anticipating the opportunity to shoot you in the face with stones when you leave the room? Is it a handicap to spend five nights in a row counting all of the tiles on the drop ceiling of your room, removing them to count the reverse side, then doing it all over countless times to check? All this because the drunken kids across the hall have spent the week throwing water under your dorm room, and banging at the door shouting obscenities. Their behavior has you so stressed that the obsessive compulsive component of Tourette syndrome is worsened. Is it a handicap to be unable to write with a pencil or pen, to rely always on a keyboard, because your hands are in perpetual motion?

Would harassment have been directed to the students in the wheelchairs? Did it happen to the blind student on campus? Would administration have allowed this to happen to them? I'm sure that the answer to these three questions is "NO!" So then I ask, "Why did it happen to me, and why was nothing done about it?"

After much reluctance by the administration to educate, and be educated, about Tourette syndrome, I decided to transfer to another, more enlightened university. Here my experience is much more positive. I have not encountered any problems in my dealings with either professors or students. Yet, interestingly, even here I have perceived a double standard.

Adam DePrince

When I am excited, anxious, nervous or upset, my tics are so exacerbated that I am often unable to speak. This necessitates a spokesperson to help me. Before my interview at my new school I typed a list of concerns and topics for my mother. She had volunteered to drive me and be my spokesperson.

In some staff members that I met at the university I sensed an aversion to the system we had developed that day to deal with the speech problem. If I were deaf would they have thought anything of my having a spokesperson? Would anyone have thought less of a wheelchair bound eighteen year old bringing a parent to help him in a totally foreign setting?

Often my tics are too severe for me to hold the telephone or to speak coherently. If I'm at home it seems the perfectly natural thing to do is to have a parent make a call for me. Especially if this call is of a professional nature. Whom should I choose to perform this service – my little brother? Yet professionals have made disdainful comments that reflect their opinion of having my mother make a telephone call for me. If I were deaf would they want to speak directly to me? Would it be so unacceptable then for my parent to make the call?

Mine is not a handicap that has drawn expositions of, "Ah, how cute . . . how sweet." This is not an attractive handicap. It is distracting and usually upsetting to others. I truly believe that with the proper knowledge the public can learn to look beyond the grunts, groans, flapping and eyerolling to the real person.

Quincy, Geraldo and *L.A. Law* were not enough. We need to be open and outspoken about Tourette syndrome. We don't want pity, but we are entitled to the same empathy that is given to the Dannys and Nancys of the world. At the same time we are entitled to be treated with the same dignity and respect as any other human being.

I, for one, do not intend to allow the misfortunes of the past to stand in my way. I am presently a second semester Freshman in college, taking mostly Junior level courses. I plan to become well known and respected in my chosen field of Computer and Information Sciences. Everyone I meet along the way will learn that people with Tourette syndrome are not crazy or weird. They are people with a handicap. They are people with potential. They are, above all, people ... with feelings.

SUBWAY PEOPLE

by

Frank Brancaccio

Mary Lou Reaver ran a call for manuscripts in the Winter 1991 Pennsylvania Tourette Syndrome Association newsletter. A week later, Frank's article arrived in my mailbox. I found myself thinking again of the incredible gift of early diagnosis and of the power with which Frank talks about his depression and isolation. It's a simple story - but also one of the most moving.

Adam Ward Seligman

It is New Year's Eve Day 1991. What a year! I turned 50 years old on September 12th, and I felt like I had recently been reborn.

I had been diagnosed with Tourette syndrome in 1975 when I was 34 years old, in New York City at the Paine

29

Whitney Clinic. I was an out patient seeing a therapist for one of my bouts of depression. I will never forget how I felt that day. I thought to myself, 'My God, I'm one of those people I see sometimes on the subway that always looked so crazy.' Leaving the hospital confused and even more depressed, I went straight home to my apartment in Greenwich Village, where I lived with a friend. When I told him, which was hard, he said, "Well at least you know what's wrong with you."

All my life everyone always thought I was a nervous wreck, but in my mind either consciously or subconsciously, I always knew I was one of the subway people, as I would call them.

Although I never screamed out profanities, I never even cursed, it's not part of my vocabulary. I had vocal tics such as grunting or sniffing. I'd be sitting at the theater and the stranger next to me would hand me a tissue. How embarrassed I would feel.

I moved to New York from Philadelphia in 1969 to study and become an actor, a dream I had all my life. This time I made the move with a friend so I had a better chance at staying. I tried moving there twice before in 1961 and 1964, but after a short time I went back to Philadelphia. I always believed in the best, so in 1961 and 1964, I studied and worked for Stella Adler, and in 1969 to 1976, with Uta Hagen and Alice Spivak. I was always one of the best actors in class. I was becoming known as a great classroom actor, but I couldn't perform outside that room. When I would go into character I would lose the tics and become someone else, but as soon as the scene ended they would be back again. I was never able to memorize lines exactly. In class, it would be mostly paraphrasing, and no one really knew or cared. But in a legitimate play the author wants his words said as he wrote them.

When I was diagnosed in 1975, my doctor treated me with Haldol and gave me literature to read. I read them and then threw them away. I couldn't deal with the subject matter. I told no one of my diagnosis except my one friend. I would rather people think I was nervous wreck then I had Tourette syndrome.

The Haldol kept being increased over a period of time, and I lost my vocal tics. With will power I was able to control the motor tics a little better. But something else started happening. In August 1976 while vacationing with friends in Provincetown, I felt real strange. I couldn't understand what was happening. All I knew was that I wanted to hide. This started a two year depression when I completely withdrew from the world. I don't think it was caused by the Haldol because I rarely get side effects. I know because I had been on so many medications at one time or another. All I knew this time is that I wanted to die, but I didn't want to kill myself. I am not a suicidal person. Needless to say this depression changed my life. It finally left me in 1978 when I made the decision to go on with my life. It was my first awakening.

I struggled along from 1978 to 1988 starting and ending abusive relationships and going from job to job. I abused charge accounts and was always looking for instant gratification.

In 1989 I moved back to Philadelphia feeling completely worthless. I went home to live with my Mother to be protected from the world. In June 1989 I started back into therapy. I didn't know what good it would do me since I had been in therapy since 1970 and I had never really changed. When I told this to my therapist, she said something no one ever said to me before, that therapy does not help without

31

support. I realized then, how can I expect people to support and understand me when I don't understand myself?

First thing I said I wanted to work on in therapy was self esteem. She then started bringing me information on Tourette syndrome and an 800 number to call for support and information. I was hesitant on doing this but she gave it to me as an assignment and I always listen to my boss.

I called the 800 number and became acquainted with a remarkable woman named Mary Lou Reaver. She told me of meetings of support groups, and she recommended books on Tourette syndrome. I started to learn so much about myself. With knowledge comes understanding. I finally understood my dysfunctional life. I also learned about my strengths.

In February 1991 I enrolled in college to get a degree in Mental Health Social Services. By the end of the year I had made the honor roll. I wanted at first to work with and counsel Tourette syndrome patients because it's so close to my heart now. But I was told by my doctors that here in Philadelphia there is no demand for this, so I began my internship in January at an AIDS clinic, knowing, however, that there is a demand and need more than just the "Subway People" lead us to believe.

I've been off Haldol for about a year now. At the present time I'm on Orap and never felt better. I still have the tics but when fellow students ask about them, I tell them I have Tourette syndrome. When I explain some of the physical and mental limitations, they laugh and say they think they have it too.

It's wonderful to be no longer afraid of the subway people, for I feel that even though I have to work a little harder than some others do, with support and knowledge I found out that I am a caring and worthwhile person, and have been blessed.

IN THE BLINK
OF AN EYE

by

Adam Ward Seligman

It's hard to believe that the order of your life can be changed in the blink of an eye.

That is what happened to me.

For me, growing up in the late 1960s, life was very sweet. At seven I was the youngest of five children, the third son of a successful Hollywood producer and his story editor wife. My father, Selig J. Seligman, had produced the television shows *Combat!, Shindig* and *Day In Court*. In 1969 he was producing motion pictures, with the help of my mother Muriel. She was responsible for his making the film *Charly*, which was to win Cliff Robertson the Academy Award in 1969 for best actor. Dad also produced the classic antiwar movie *Hell in the Pacific*.

My two older brothers were aspiring writers; Joel had just

started college, and Brad was the National High School Debate Champion in 1969. My sister, Dale, was studying voice and rebellion, and Lucy, five years older than me, was going through the throes of pre-adolescence and making my life hell (her duty as an older sister!) Over all I was happy, despite some speech problems that were being modified by tutoring.

Then, one summer night, everything changed.

My father died unexpectedly in his sleep at the age of fifty - one. It was the night Brad won the debate Nationals and my parents had been at a screening. My father was elated when he came home and before going to sleep, had spoken proudly of his children to my mother. Then he died. My mother was in a state of shock, with five children to raise. She had never been on her own before. Dale and Joel stepped in and tried to get the family together. But it was difficult. Joel moved back to Los Angeles from Berkeley to go to UCLA, and Dale spent most of the summer with Mom.

Lucy and I were sent to summer camp so our mother could deal with the new responsibilities that had suddenly befallen her. I wandered the camp in a daze, bewildered and confused, not totally tuned into my new life. I felt profound grief, but, at seven, was unsure how to show it. It would be years before I could cry about my father's death, and even then the tears were hard to come by. Crying never came easy to me; especially crying about my own pain. I could cry for my mother, for friends grieving, but something inside me didn't allow sympathy for myself.

One day I came into the bunkhouse and found another camper sprawled on my bunk. I asked him to move. He began making faces at me — blinking his eyes, shrugging his shoulders and smacking his lips.

"Why are you doing that?" I demanded.

"That's what you do — ALL THE TIME!" he said. I punched him in the stomach, one of the only times in my life that

I have been violent. Then I looked in a mirror.

He was right.

My eyes were blinking out of control. I tried to stop them and realized that I had been blinking for several days without paying much attention to it. My neck itched inside. I felt a strange sensation in my neck and shoulder muscles that could only be relieved by twitching them — a shrugging movement that became over time a sharp jerking. I made soft kissing noises and felt a weird sensation in my throat. I wanted to make more noises, sounds, but I stopped myself.

When I received a postcard from mother that she had to give away our dog Alex, I found to my horror that the sensation in my throat was a desire to bark. I tried to control it but the other boys in the bunk house noticed it and made fun of me. This was my first experience with teasing. It wouldn't be my last. I wanted to go home but I couldn't. I stayed in my bunk, reading by myself and trying to figure out what was wrong with me. I had no idea.

When camp ended and I went home, Mom noticed the blinking and noises and asked me to stop. I told her that I couldn't stop them. Over the next few months my facial tics and noises changed rapidly. My arms and then my legs became affected. I began shaking my left wrist, making kicking motions, stamping, rubbing the front of my sneakers so often that I ruined a new pair in less than a week. Nobody could figure out what to do.

I use the word tic or twitch with a very strong sense of the difference. A tic, to me, was a rapid uncontrolled involuntary movement of a small range; an eye blinking, a grimace, a small jerk of the hand. A twitch was what my neck did several times a minute; a violent large movement that quite often produced pain and had an internal feeling proceeding it, a sense of energy building up that had to be released by movement. The neck twitch, or the larger body movements were what I called twitches. Everything else I called a tic, including the noises that felt similar to a tic internally.

My family, as always, responded with gentle humor. If I were going to tic and make noises, they weren't going to make too big a deal of it. The running joke around the dinner table became, "What's the tic of the week?" They weren't insensitive, just not willing to pay too much attention to my odd behavior.

When I had a lengthy episode of hallucinations at eight, my family began paying more serious attention. While watching television one night, I saw my father's face appear on the screen, then a swarm of insects shot out of it. I had a thorough work up at Children's Hospital in Hollywood, with psychological, neurological and physical exams. I had an EEG and blood tests. The tests all came back normal. The diagnosis was 'separation anxiety,' a perfectly valid psychiatric diagnosis. I began seeing a child psychiatrist at the age of eight for four sessions a week. "Obviously," said the psychiatrist, "the shock of losing your father is causing your tics and noises." So, it was assumed that after eighteen months or so of analysis things would get better.

They didn't.

At the age of nine I was watching my brother, Brad, play ping pong with our family friend J.B. I was sitting, eyes blinking, neck jerking and making my usual barking noises. J.B. missed a shot and swore. Well, by the next day that had become my word, my new vocal tic. Things didn't seem funny at all anymore to my family. My brother, Joel, spoke to my psychiatrist who assured him it was only another symptom of the deep anger I was feeling due to my father's death, and not to worry. Only my family did.

The thing that was interesting about the swearing is that at first it felt like a physical tic; involuntary, uncontrolled, rapid. But soon it built up into a stronger feeling of internal tension, more like the feeling in my neck but less violent. Often just saying the swear word softly relieved the urge. Other times it came out explosively; a bark or a shout. Always, it shocked people or stunned them when they realized what I was saying.

In 1971 my grandfather had a stroke and while my mother was in New York with him, I underwent extensive psychological testing at the public school I was attending. Their diagnosis was that I was suffering from mild psychosis. I was kicked out of school for fear I was dangerous. The teachers didn't want me in their classrooms swearing at them. The other students made fun of me so I accepted the diagnosis as perfectly understandable — everyone at school said I was crazy, so I must be. I became increasingly reclusive, missing class after class due to the fear of being teased. I remember walking home the day I was expelled, almost relieved by the thought that no longer would I have to explain to the other students that I was a Martian and the tics were how I communicated. At home that day I curled up with a book and grunted to myself, neck twitching, foot jerking.

My mother enrolled me in a private therapeutic school called Park Century. It was incredibly expensive, as were the psychiatrist and the medications I took. Luckily, the state paid for some of my tuition because I was considered Seriously Emotionally Disturbed; S.E.D.

It was the third label I had been given in less than a year.

During the next few year's life took on an unreal tinge. My tics changed over time, with new tics replacing old ones about every three months. My vocal tics also changed, with the swearing stopping completely at age eleven only to be replaced by a series of grunts, barks, and smacking noises. One year I had spitting tics. Another time I chewed obsessively on the left collar of my shirt. I had tics in the stomach, making motions of my diaphragm. I had nightmares and hallucinations every few months.

Why the tics changed, or even existed at all, I didn't know. But over time, slowly, so slowly, I gained an awareness of my body. I could tell sometimes before a very severe tic that it was going to happen. If it were a noise, I would tighten up my stomach and try to suppress it. Other times I would let the tic out, hoping to satisfy the inner urge to grunt or twitch.

I was on a series of medications, including haloperidol, which was supposed to stop tics, but in my case it caused extensive sedation. I was also on Valium for my sleep disturbance, and I was taking aspirin daily for neck pains. I saw my pediatrician weekly for neck massages and later began seeing a chiropractor.

These were the external realities of my life. There were others. The teasing on the bus from other kids, the time I was asked to leave a near empty movie theater because of my noises, the fear I had of going to public places. One thing I spoke little about, but was constant, was the pain in my neck and headaches. I feared the damage my twitches might be causing to my spine. My posture was affected by my symptoms and the stress on my stomach of suppressing tics made it difficult to stand straight.

My internal life during this time is almost totally blank to me. I have for the most part blocked it out. I don't recall much of anything from age nine to age fourteen. I know I was depressed most of the time; I felt ugly; I hated myself. But specific details escape me. I had no friends until age thirteen, no girls who liked me until fifteen. I was different — what an easy word that is for my condition! I felt safer not having any close relationships. I probably didn't want any. The people whom I loved, like my father, died, or like my brothers moved away. It was much easier not to love or to commit to a relationship of any kind. My dog Ali, was one of the only living things I felt safe around. Of course she couldn't talk, or tease me, or question me so she was the perfect companion. I could abuse her, hold her nose, wrestle with her, and she wouldn't complain. She would just lick my face and bark happily at her weird master.

The one close relationship I did have was with my mother. She always believed in me, and would reassure me that I wasn't going to be this way the rest of my life. She would tell me that I wasn't crazy, that there was something physically wrong with me, and one day we would find out what it was. She protected me from the angry looks of strangers and fought for me against my sisters. They had trouble with the amount of attention I was getting from Mom. But, most of all she loved me with no conditions, tics and all. My one friend during this period was Matt Asner. We met at school, and when I moved from there to a special education school the next year, he followed. We both were *Star Trek* fans, Trekkies, and it influenced our lives. If nothing else is true about *Star Trek*, there is the fact that Captain Kirk's best friend is 'different,' an alien from the planet Vulcan. I identified with the logical Mister Spock by repressing my emotions like he tried to in the show. Matt was the emotional one in our friendship — the Starship Captain — and was always willing to act out a feeling. Matt became a movie nut, and followed in his father's footsteps by becoming an actor. I became a science fiction fan and at thirteen started writing and submitting stories to the pulp magazines.

I was already displaying beyond average skills in English, and the combination of my tics, noises and literary ambitions seemed an odd one to my brother Joel, who had started to wonder if there was more going on than 'separation anxiety.' In 1976 when I was fourteen, he read a magazine article on a reportedly rare neurological disorder and sent it my mother. She was intrigued and told my psychiatrist about it. He seemed unimpressed and I continued therapy four times a week.

I enrolled in drama class at high school and found a new freedom in acting. The drama teacher accepted me, unlike some teachers who had not, disruptive noises and all. The first play I was in had only six characters and I won one of the parts. It was interesting to act before a group of strangers and have people compliment me on my character's tics!

I found that when I was absorbed in a scene I didn't have as many symptoms, and I was slowly learning to control or suppress the intensity of my noises then. It seemed related to breathing, this growing control, and drama class often focused on breath relaxation techniques.

When Matt joined the drama class, we began years of improvisations and scene study that led to Matt starring in the school play four years running. One year the play was *Flowers For Algernon* based on the same story as my father's movie *Charly*. On opening night the cast dedicated the show to my Dad. I chose not to inhibit my symptoms that night and they added to my characters richness, by giving him an unspoken reason to be a neurologist.

I started to notice girls when I was fourteen. My first crush was on my teacher, Karen. After a few months I started to hang out with a younger girl, Theresa, and her sister Lisa. They tolerated me but didn't quite understand what was wrong with me. I finally got the nerve to ask Theresa out. She said no and I felt crushed.

In June, 1976, my psychiatrist told me casually that he thought I had something called Tourette syndrome. It was the same disorder discussed in the magazine article Joel had read. The medication that I was taking was the recommended treatment. We gradually came to realize that he had known I had Tourette syndrome for some time, but for reasons unclear to us, didn't tell the family. I went home all excited and told my mother I had a disease, that I wasn't crazy.

"What disease?" She asked.

"I don't know — something with a French name." I responded.

Over the next few days we researched Tourette syndrome. As we learned I had a classic case: It had started between the ages of two and fourteen (the average ages of onset); I had multiple tics and involuntary vocalizations; I could control them for brief periods of time. The tics had started in my face with eye blinking and had worked down my body over time; I responded to medication.

The diagnosis made sense. That summer I became aware that, while I had many problems, I was not mentally ill. I am disabled by a neurological disorder that is caused by an imbalance of the brain chemical, dopamine, in the part of the brain that controls motor and vocal inhibition.

I remember a bus ride after my diagnosis. I was sitting on the bus, barking to myself, with my neck twitching. Two teenage girls were sitting behind me and teasing me. I finally said to one of them, "I can't help it; I have a neurological disorder."

"I have neurological hearing," she responded. "So shut up." Obviously the diagnosis wasn't going to end the teasing.

There were some atypical aspects too. My episodes of hallucinations would not be explained for close to fifteen more years. But they seemed caused by the intense sleep deprivation caused by my neck twitching. Sleep disturbance and night terrors are common in people with Tourette syndrome. The sleep disorder I had — *hypnogogic phenomena,* a form of dreams while awake, was unusual.

The timing of my father's death and the onset of my Tourette syndrome, with the resulting seven years of misdiagnosis, has always troubled me. Fortunately, in recent years doctors have begun looking into triggering factors, things that might bring out Tourette syndrome in people genetically predisposed to having it.

For instance, in my family, my grandfather had a moderate case of Tourette syndrome that lasted over eighty years without being correctly diagnosed. My brothers had facial tics and one brother had neck tics and made occasional vocalizations. These milder forms are genetically linked to Tourette syndrome.

I had a new tic in 1976, a lip smacking that was turning into a movement of my lower lip over my teeth. Because of this tic, I had frequent cuts in my mouth and sometimes these turned into cold sores. I saw the dentist frequently and was told these were normal, nothing to worry about. My orthodontist advised my mother not to fit me with braces because of the tearing in my lower lip. The braces probably would rip my gums more. As a result I grew up with badly adjusted teeth.

The summer following my diagnosis was a hectic one. We found out about the Tourette Syndrome Association, a non profit voluntary health agency based in Bayside, New York. It was founded by six families in New York City. My mother's and my life were to become closely intertwined with the organization over the next fifteen years. Soon after my mother first spoke to the Tourette Syndrome Association, she was asked to call a film maker, Dr. Barnett Addis, at the Neuro Psychiatric Institute at UCLA. He was making a documentary film about Tourette syndrome and mother was asked to be his liaison with the Tourette Syndrome Association.

Dr. Addis was the first person I had met who had any real knowledge of Tourette syndrome. He had interviewed people with Tourette syndrome from all over the country and he showed me footage of some of the people. One young college student, Orrin, had severe tics and vocalizations including obscenities. He was shown playing guitar in his dorm room and sitting in a classroom, his tics presented as part of the total picture. I found him awe inspiring.

The film crew filmed me briefly that summer and the film they made, *The Sudden Intruder,* would go on to win awards and be shown on PBS for years. It helped diagnose hundreds of cases. It also helped educate doctors with what was then sketchy knowledge of what Tourette syndrome was and how to treat it.

After I was diagnosed, the real problems began. The major

issues were education and medication.

In the area of education I was still receiving special help as S.E.D. We spent the next few years trying to get this changed to Other Physical Impairment, a less loaded label. Because I was the first known case of Tourette syndrome in my school district and had been funded for several years, the special education panel decided they wanted to meet me. During my last three years of high school, I met with members of the Board of Education twice a year trying to educate them and to work out my Individual Education Plan, or an I.E.P. I was finally classified as Other Health Impaired.

Now, thanks to Public Law 94-142, The Education for all Handicapped Children Act, this process, once the diagnosis and placement are worked through, is easier for parents to muddle through. But in the mid to late 1970's disabled children were treated on a case – by – case basis and I had no guarantee of receiving funding each year. The school I attended was expensive. Due to my years of misdiagnosis, and my sister Lucy's accident at a folk dance coffeehouse, my mother had spent a large portion of my father's estate on medical expenses. For me education expenses were now covered, but for many families getting the help that is their right under Federal Law remains a nightmare.

Medication now became the major problem. Before I was diagnosed I was treated with Haloperidol, a very potent antipsychotic medication that initially was the drug of choice for Tourette syndrome in this country. It blocks dopamine receptors in the brain, thereby reducing tics. But it also causes dry mouth, appetite gain, excessive thirst, depression, fatigue and sedation. It became apparent in 1976 that another treatment plan would have to be found.

I tried close to thirty medications over the next three years. These ranged from drugs chemically similar to Haldol, to drugs for seizures, migraines, manic depression and some experimental medications. I became a professional 'guinea pig.' All of the medications had severe side effects, and my grades began to drop accordingly. In my senior year of high school I was told I would have to retake close to a year of classes because of incomplete grades. As a result I couldn't graduate with my class. I was devastated, and my subsequent problems with college and work seem based on that terrible blow to my self esteem.

Theresa's step sister, Tina, entered my class that year and I found myself hanging out with her a lot, eating ice cream cones at the park where we had P.E. and sitting next to her in class. I asked her out and to my amazement she said yes! We planned a double date with my sister and her husband.

The date was awkward, probably because Tina was less naive about life than I was. But after dancing to records in my sister's living room, we sat on the couch and she introduced me to kissing. It was great, although the neck twitches made me lurch backwards every so often. Once I fell off the couch and she laughed at the situation, not at me. I fell in love.

My lower lip had developed a permanent lesion and it became apparent that a combination of surgery and severely increased medication would be needed. I spent three days in the hospital, on an intravenous drip of Haldol and in constant pain from the sutures, which triggered mouth tics. But it healed and I never had that problem again.

When people try to give me the reassuring line that at least I wasn't in a wheelchair, or blind, as though my pain was lessened by not having those disabilities, I grow angry. I don't think you can compare pain the way you can compare cars. Tourette syndrome is not an economy model; in fact, it may be the Rolls Royce of embarrassing and emotionally painful neurological disorders.

In the late 1970's I met Orrin, the college student from the film, who impressed me so when he visited Los Angeles. Although he was older than me, we got along well. I found a new strength in knowing somebody else with Tourette syndrome. He was to become my first 'brother in Tourette' and over the years we've stayed in touch. In 1980 while visiting New York, we were thrown out of cafes together for our noises. It was an exhilarating experience. Orrin went on to become a psychiatrist and a Board Director of the Tourette Syndrome Association. He remains one of my closest friends.

In 1990 we were interviewed together on *Geraldo*. After the show we traded survival stories for hours. I also had a therapy session with him and began to deal with Tourette syndrome from a new point of view — that of a chronic lifelong disorder that I had to learn to live with.

In 1979, my final year in high school, a friend of ours at the Tourette Syndrome Association told us about a drug called pimozide. It was highly effective in treating Tourette syndrome, was milder than Haldol, and had fewer side effects. There was a catch; although it had been used in Europe since the late 1950's it wasn't available in the United States. My mother decided to smuggle it in from Canada and France.

I started taking low doses of pimozide in the Spring of 1979. The results were impressive, and the side effects were much less severe than Haldol. When I was seventeen and realized that I wasn't going to graduate, I dropped out of school for a few months to get used to the medication and to fulfill a life long dream — I went on an archaeological dig.

The Canyon Pintado site in Western Colorado and Utah was being surveyed and excavated by the University of Colorado, Fort Collins. I joined the summer class there in May of 1979 and spent three weeks learning about archaeology and the history of the Arapaho culture.

It was my first experience with peers older than myself and

I quickly found myself fitting in, in a way that was different from my experience with high school students. Older people, in this case college students, seemed more willing to accept me. They were also more willing to get me drunk and their friendship, long days and constant beer drinking did wonders for my self esteem. My Tourette syndrome was quieter then, but after six weeks of heat and intense exhaustion, my cursing came back very severely. In the eighth week of the program I decided to go home and find out more about this symptom. I said good-bye to my friends on the dig, paid one last visit to some of the rock art in Rangely, and flew home.

I discovered that coprolalia – involuntary cursing – affected up to a third of people with Tourette syndrome. It appears to be similar to post stroke language behavior and this implies an organic etiology. The theory I grew to accept in the 1980's was that there was a separate language center in the brain, a 'bad word box,' and that when a disorder of inhibition like Tourette syndrome developed, the inhibitions went away. The fact that I was saying words with a heavy sexual content was ignored through my years of therapy, but it deeply affected my sex life. Very few women want to go out with man as 'blunt' as me, and the women I did get involved with, until recently, were very bad for me. I had to learn to accept my sexuality and my cursing, and in the process I gained new confidence.

I dated a young woman with Tourette syndrome at this point who went to the same doctor. Her symptoms were milder than mine and her fear of seeing my more severe symptoms drove her away. I realized that it wasn't enough for a couple to share Tourette syndrome. They had to share the courage of being together despite symptom level.

Many friends have assumed that I would be happiest with another person with Tourette syndrome. While I have dated women with and without Tourette syndrome, I find the differences have little to do with the experience of disability. I have met women who don't have Tourette syndrome who were more accepting of me, and women with Tourette syndrome with severe prejudices. What I have learned is that people are more than just a collection of symptoms — they are the total of all they have experienced and learned in their lives.

In later years, again while on an archaeological dig, this time in Israel, I redeveloped involuntary spitting. This combination of symptoms — tics of the face and left hand, neck jerking, cursing and spitting, has been the same with changes in intensity over the last ten years. It has made life humiliating at times, but also has brought new challenges to living that I would not give up. I realize now that being disabled is not a bad thing. The social stigma attached to it is still high, but awareness of the disabled among the general population grew a lot in the 1980's and I was an integral part of this new awareness.

In June, 1980 I happily graduated high school, a year later than my peers, but still a goal I hadn't been sure I would meet. The next day the phone rang. It was Abbey Meyer, the Director of Patient Services at the Tourette Syndrome Association, and a good friend of the family. My mother spoke with her for a few minutes and then turned to me. She said, "They want me to testify before Congress about the trouble we've had getting pimozide. I can't do that."

"I'll go." I said boldly, having little idea of what was involved. Abbey was delighted and I flew to Washington D.C. three days later to testify. I met several of the then small Rare Disorder lobby or what the media called 'Orphan' disorders. Orphan meant that the number of people affected was so small that no pharmaceutical house, for financial reasons, would adopt the disease to research and hopefully to treat. Orphan disorders range from myoclonus with fewer than 1,000 cases in the United States to Parkinson's Disease that affects large numbers. I was in exciting company. Marjorie Guthrie, the feisty widow of folk singer Woody Guthrie, who died in a state institution with Huntington's Chorea, was the patron saint of the rare disorder lobby. Along with Abbey and a young woman with myoclonus, I spoke to a panel of thirteen Congressional Representatives that summer morning.

Afterwards I was interviewed by a young reporter from the Los Angeles Times. Two days later a short piece about my testimony ran in the front section. Shortly after that I was contacted by Maurice Klugman, the brother of actor Jack Klugman, and Associate Producer on the *Quincy* television show.

"We want to do an episode on Tourette syndrome and the Orphan Drug issue," he told me. That began an exchange and in November Sam Egan a writer — producer of *Quincy*, called me.

They were to film in January and Sam offered me the position of Technical Advisor on that episode. I worked on the script checking for accuracy and met several times with the show's medical consultant, Mark Taylor, a former coroner. The very talented actor Paul Clemmons got the part of the Tourette syndrome patient who goes to Washington in the wake of his friend's accidental death. I worked daily with him for ten days teaching him my symptoms and trading jokes. Paul called my lessons, "the tics of the trade!"

I remember sitting on the set one afternoon when the story editor called a meeting. "We need to write a scene about side effects. If we just have the character go off his medicine without an explanation, we'll get complaints." Sam Egan, the story editor and I sat down with a legal pad. Thirty minutes later the three of us had drafted a scene. It was typed up and filmed the next morning. That was my first experience writing for television and I was hooked. I felt proud that the show's staff trusted me enough to include my input in this crucial sequence of the story.

After the filming of that episode I met with the story editors of *Quincy* and sold them an original story. I was then able to join the Writers Guild of America, becoming the youngest current member at that time. After that I sold several scenes to a comedy series on cable, and found myself with an agent and what I thought would be a career in free-lance television writing.

I was wrong of course. To work in Hollywood requires selling yourself. At 18, with little self confidence and an obvious disability, I was a difficult sell. I felt my agent didn't try very hard and although I took screenwriting classes and creative writing workshops, my writing didn't jump out at you and scream "Buy me!" to Hollywood. After a couple of years of this struggle I realized that paying my dues would be required; I would need more life experience before I could write for a living.

The *Quincy* episode aired that Spring. The media attention on both Tourette syndrome and the orphan drug issue had many ramifications. First, hundreds of people with Tourette syndrome were diagnosed. This number has increased to thousands over ten years of reruns. Second, the Orphan Drug Act was revived in Congress and the rare disease lobby began an intensive campaign to get legislation passed. In 1981 I flew to Washington D.C. with Jack Klugman and we testified before a packed chamber of Congress.

The following year *Quincy* did a follow up episode about the orphan drug issue and featured the disorder myoclonus. My friend from the hearing flew out to advise the show. My mother cast five hundred people with rare disorders for a fictional march on Washington D.C. for the episode.

That was the year I went back to college. As I look back on my college years from 1980 to 1985, they seem frustrating. But, during those years I grew in many ways, both as a person and as a writer. I did well in my grades, but the ever present duo of symptoms and side effects from the medication were with me constantly. Incomplete classes marred my last year at Loyola

Adam Ward Seligman

Marymount University.

I moved away from home in 1983 first to campus housing and later to a two bedroom apartment in Santa Monica. Living on my own was difficult; I missed the support of my mother and I found the solitude depressing. I was often depressed and occasionally suicidal. After I moved to Santa Monica, my friend Matt lived with me. While we were, and still are, compatible as friends, as room mates we were a disaster. It is strange how being the best of friends leaves you ill prepared to working out living differences. We argued about music, food, cleaning duties and fought over using the phone.

New Years morning, 1986, found the two of us in an all night cafe snorting cocaine with two women we had met. Matt was recovering from addiction and I felt terrible that I had been involved in what might have been a return to drug abuse. As it turned out, it was the last time he used. I, on the other hand, would add it to my list of addictions in the 1990's

After that my dear friend from college, Suzanne Madison, moved in with me for two years. She complained about my apparent need to not clean the bathroom every five minutes, but she proved to be a good friend and housemate. Like most of the women I get along with, I found myself in love with her, but in this situation I was able to control my need to tell her. She sensed something, but her boyfriend kept things cool.

When I attended college, I usually met my professors before the semester began to introduce them to Tourette syndrome. I also explained it to the class at the first meeting. This had interesting results. In one class a young woman pointedly moved away from me before class began, making several rude comments. By the end of the semester we had become friends and even dated!

That date was a learning experience of the negative kind. I picked Cindy up, and we went to dinner at a nice French restaurant and talked over wine. Then we went to a screening at the Writers Guild. You might call this a typical Hollywood writers evening out.

Only I wasn't a typical Hollywood writer. Throughout the evening I had excessive tics and vocalizations, and was repeatedly stared at. During the movie we had to move several times, People made comments to the guard. Cindy grew more uncomfortable and afterwards asked to be taken home. We remained friends, but obviously there was more to going out with me than just a date: I brought my disease with me.

My spiritual mother at college was Pat Oliver, a wonderful speech professor who also advised the campus newspaper. She quickly had me writing and speaking out with increasing frequency. When she taught women's studies it seemed natural for me to attend the class. As one of two men among thirty women, my Tourette syndrome stood out even more as we discussed issues of reproductive freedom, date rape and the woman's movement. I met my closest friends at Loyola Marymount University in that class. It helped to open me up politically and I was able to look beyond disability politics to civil rights for everyone.

My brother, Brad, practiced civil rights law in Oakland. In discussions with him about my life I had a growing sense that Los Angeles, college and television writing were not the right life style for me.

It seemed that every few months I took off North to Big Sur, Berkeley and Monterey, searching for something. I sensed that John Steinbeck knew what it was. I devoured his books while sitting at Nepenthe, brandied coffee in hand. It wasn't a place but a philosophy that I came to discover.

In their book *The Log From the Sea of Cortez*, Steinbeck and his friend Ed Ricketts discuss cause and effect thinking and consider the alternative, nonteleological thinking; 'IS thinking.'

Instead of blaming things, for instance my disability, for events I had no control over – my father's death, my grandfathers genes – I looked at what is, not what was. In nonteleological terms this became the search for not why things occur but an acceptance of what is. I had Tourette syndrome — now what? The answer was slowly coming to me as I lived out the lives of a college student, a free-lance writer, a disability rights advocate, a lonely man. The answer seemed in finding a community and world I could belong to.

I seemed to have found it when I began working as a publicist for a small jazz record label in 1987. Working with the musicians I loved, helping them get record deals, talking to editors and music writers across the country was a delightful trip into an aspect of the entertainment business with which I had no previous experience. It also proved to be increasingly stressful as my symptoms worsened over the next two and a half years, and I developed some strange fixations and recurring thoughts that didn't seem associated with Tourette syndrome.

In November of 1987 I went to Chicago to address the American Medical Writers Association on Tourette syndrome. I made a successful and moving presentation. The next day I flew to Cincinnati for the Tourette Syndrome Association Leadership Conference. On the airplane I sat alone, twitching away, and reading science fiction writer Robert Silverberg. Looking up as the plane was boarding, I saw a young woman gazing at me intensely. Oh hell, I thought. Here come the questions.

"Are you going to the Tourette conference," She asked cheerfully. As she did so she blinked several times.

"Yes. Are you?"

"Uh huh. You were in that film, weren't you?"

I invited her to sit and over the next hour got to know her. Eli was seventeen, a high school senior and this was her first conference too. She was obviously holding in her tics but how much so I didn't know until later when she lost her ability to suppress midway through the conference, exploding with tics and noises. She was delightful to talk to and confessed that she had watched my part of the film repeatedly when her symptoms were severe.

It was at the Tourette Syndrome Conference that my search for community ended. Within a few hours a dozen adults with Tourette syndrome, ranging from mild cases like the spunky president of the Florida chapter to the very severe president of the Boston chapter, had come together and were holding an all Tourette table at dinner. Joining us were writer Oliver Sacks, and photographer Lowell Handler who had collaborated on a piece for Life Magazine that came out in 1988. In talking to Lowell that evening I described the weird intrusive thoughts of violence, suicide and sex that were interfering with my concentration at work. He listened closely, then to my amazement told me that he had similar obsessions.

Obsessive Compulsive Disorder was a new term to me but as I grew to know more about it, I realized that I had it all my life. Closely related to Tourette syndrome genetically, it manifested itself as thoughts or compulsive acts that like Tourette syndrome could not be controlled. In reading Judith Rappaport's book *The Boy Who Couldn't Stop Washing* there are multiple references to Obsessive Compulsive Disorder and Tourette syndrome.

On the lighter side, I developed an infatuation with one woman, a deep friendship with the President of the Boston Chapter, and a brother /sister relationship with Eli. As the conference grew to a close we discussed holding a Tourette syndrome retreat for the 'Adult Group' as we had grown to be called by people at the Tourette Syndrome Association.

The retreat happened in April of 1990. I had finally broken free of Los Angeles and had moved North to Berkeley near my brother Brad. I was working on a novel about Tourette syndrome, consulting with television shows and writing articles for the three leading drum magazines. When I flew to Chicago I was met by Eli, no longer a kid but a woman, and another young man with Tourette syndrome and severe Obsessive Compulsive Disorder. We drove to the Ozarks where the others were waiting for us. Over the next three days we lived the life of a Tourette community where the only time tics were commented on was when they struck the collective funny bone of the group. My friend Orrin and I played music every night; we all sang Beatles songs and drank far too much, but it was the closest and warmest weekend I have ever spent.

The year 1990 was pivotal for me. Besides the retreat, I also was involved in three relationships of varying intensity that both helped my self esteem and suggested to me that emotionally I still had much growing to do. Throughout the year I worked on a novel about Tourette syndrome called *Echolalia*, which centered me for most of the year. As the year progressed and I got used to living alone, I found myself ending every evening by drinking a few beers or a bottle of wine. By years end I realized that I was becoming an alcoholic.

The relationship between alcoholism and disability is a strong one. Living lives of solitude, rejection and sometimes frightening medical crisis, often disabled people turn to substance abuse. I had talked about this once with a social worker, years before. My neurologist commented that I was using alcohol to turn off my brain at night, drinking myself to sleep. He also told me that my increase in symptoms was probably related to the damage the alcohol was doing to my system.

Still I drank. I realized that since 1979 when I was on the archaeological dig I had drunk often to relax. Somewhere over the years the fun of drinking with people at concerts or at parties had somehow changed into the fun of just drinking. Only it wasn't fun anymore. It was something I had to do. Sometimes as the day ended I would check the kitchen for beer, wine, scotch, try to get some marijuana, make sure I had sleeping pills in case none of these worked to knock me out. I didn't have black outs: I just drank myself to sleep. I didn't have a drinking problem: I just drank every day.

I stopped drinking daily at the beginning of 1991 and probably will always have a problem with alcohol. I sleep better without it, and yes, my Tourette syndrome symptoms are much reduced without it. I go to Alcoholics Anonymous and try to work the steps. I don't fully understand the idea of a 'higher power' and when I try to relate to it, I think of my writing muse, the force that allows me to create no matter what happens in my life. My muse is fueled by my deep friendships with the Tourette syndrome community, and my new friends at Alcoholics Anonymous.

My novel *Echolalia* was accepted for publication and came out in the summer of 1991 by Hope Press, an all Tourette syndrome oriented publishing house. After fifteen years of writing, I had succeeded in my goals: I had a place to live, a family who loved me, and a published novel.

I also still have Tourette syndrome. But it doesn't have me. This may be the best lesson I have learned in my life. I hope it isn't the only one.

In The Blink Of An Eye was written for an audio cassette in 1991. It was edited with the loving attention of my producer Neva Duyndam. It is available on cassette (51 minutes in length) from: Duvall Media, Inc. P.O. Box 15892, Newport Beach, CA. 92659. The cost is $9.95 plus $2.00 Shipping and handling. To order by phone call (800) 726-3465. Duvall Media Inc has other Tourette syndrome related tapes. For a catalog call (714) 631-3445.

Adam Ward Seligman

IN WALKED MAURA

by

Maura Woodruff

I was laying in a hospital bed, IV in place. I had donated my spinal fluid, urine, and blood, and had made a video study of my tics and vocalizations. I had made personal disclosures to a host of psychiatric and family history questions as well. The neurological tests were all in the name of Tourette syndrome research. (In spite of my generosity, they still want my brain! I did agree to that, but only when I'm done with it.) One of my evaluators told me of someone who was also participating in the study but had never met anyone else with Tourette syndrome. He said that she would like to meet me. I had no problem with that and in walked Maura. We talked for a couple of hours, with little of that time devoted to Tourette syndrome. She is a biology major. I am a science teacher. We both have Tourette syndrome yet we spoke mostly of spirituality and our experiences of the divine. Her depth and maturity of spirit, her poignant insights, her intelligence, her

57

soul-rattling poetry, moved me to believe that she could be one of my teachers. She was the first woman with Tourette syndrome I had ever met. Thus the reflections of myself and my Tourette syndrome I would perceive in her would differ from that of the many Tourette syndrome males I know.

Maura is intense. The reader will garner that from her writings.

"Maura, I really want your contribution to our book," I told her. "I can't write," she said. "Your poetry betrays that untruth." "Oh, I can write that, but not 'my autobiography'." "Then write about your poetry." She did and both her poetry, born out from her pain and struggles and her commentary are testimony to her intense and provocative spirit. "Intensity" is a good character-ization of the Tourette syndrome experience, for our tics are intense, as our other symptoms and our contemplations and lives, our play and stories, and our effect on others. And Maura does us all a great service in ably communicating the intensity that animates us.

John S. Hilkevich

Don't you know me? I sat next to you in the fourth grade. I was the shy one. The girl who everyone watched with fear. Others snickered while I sat there, jerking my arms and legs uncontrol-lably. I always made them laugh, as my face distorted into many expressions, as if I were telling a joke, to coincide with the occasional noises that would creep out of me. It's me, Maura Woodruff. I remember you watching me, looking as if you had something to say; yet you always remained quiet and stared with gleaming eyes. Don't you know me, or were you too afraid because you didn't understand me? Well, I didn't understand me either; until now.

The fourth grade was hard for me. It was when I was first diagnosed as having Tourette syndrome. Somehow, without fully understanding why, I felt as if I had plummeted into a new world where I had no control. It seemed as if I were dead, and someone else had complete control over my body, yet I was still very aware of my surroundings. The pain shot through me like a dagger, when the kids would ridicule me and walk away. Many of my friends from that moment on had left me. Even those few that had remained at the time, eventually went their separate ways. I then realized that I was alone in this fight against myself. In order for others to understand me, I must first understand myself. This is where my battle began.

I spent Halloween week in the hospital upon diagnosis. I was administered the medication clonidine on a trial basis, and eventually used it as a form of treatment for my tics. It seemed to work well on my tics, but the side effects became a hassle. My blood pressure continually dropped. I became so lethargic that I slept most of the time. I also found it hard to concentrate, as I became paranoid about everything.

Two years later, I again went to the hospital where they conducted many tests and put me on Haldol, while weaning me off Clonidine. This was a trip and a half as the two medications peaked at different times. I went from being lethargic to overly excited often throughout the course of the day. Eventually, I was on Haldol alone.

The sixth grade was the hardest for me. My tics were at their worst during the next two years. I was constantly sniffing, coughing and clearing my throat. Sometimes I got the hiccups for hours and would grunt and whine occasionally. It seemed that no matter how hard I tried, I could not sit still. I even burst out laughing sometimes for no apparent reason. I was too disruptive in class and that made learning more difficult for me and the kids who sat by me. I was always a good student, just difficult to understand.

After a few months of taking low doses of Haldol to no avail, they started to increase the dosage. This is where the trouble began. At first I started to get body tremors, and since the doctors didn't deem it harmful and my tics still hadn't subsided we increased the dosage again. Since the first day of increased dosage there was trouble. I had a full fledged seizure that at first came on slowly, where my leg muscles became stiff so I could not move them and my jaw locked. When I went to sit, my eyes rolled back into my head and my body began to convulse. It was a frightening experience as I didn't understand what was happening to me, and I thought I might even die! My parents rushed me to the emergency room where we waited for hours, while I suffered painful muscle contractions. When I started experiencing difficulty breathing, they immediately administered Cogentin to counteract the side effects. Afterward, I continually played with the dosage of Haldol, but could not find a happy medium. I ended up taking Cogentin whenever I had a reaction because of the Haldol, which was at least once a week.

The frequent reactions were very painful and scared many people away. I began to feel isolated as my friends could not understand the new me. Things at home were not great either. There was constant rivalry among my siblings as they began to hate every aspect of my life. They hated what they perceived to be 'over protectiveness' from my parents. I hated them because it seemed as if they were allowed to do things and I wasn't. I was always being yelled at to be quiet or sit still. I guess since I was on the medication it was thought that there was no excuse for the way I was acting. They believed I was just faking it to get attention. I never understood this logic. Why would someone fake something that was both terrifying and painful? Didn't they understand me at all? Even now, it is still denied when the subject is brought up. I could see the pain in my father's eyes, looking as if he were asking what he did to deserve a child like me. He always made it clear (in my perception), that my presence was not wanted. This is very hard for me to accept even now.

The following represents some of the pain I felt because of lost friends, as well as the fear of gaining new ones whom I thought would eventually go away. This is how I perceived myself then, and sometimes even now.

> I can no longer fight the pain within me
> It's a battle never to be won.
> As I twist and turn, my body moves crazily
> Scaring off friends who have yet to come.
> Alone and afraid I go my way
> As my heart is always betrayed.
> I can no longer see the life before me
> For now I live in the past.
> I struggle to see a better way
> But nothing remains in sight.
> It's a battle of wits
> A battle of soul,
> A battle I cannot fight.
> Pain and loneliness are the victors
> For they always rule my life.
> Alone in a crowd I shall always be
> For I am a horrible sight.

The doctors were discussing the new medication, pimozide, with my mother when I entered the eighth grade. They decided to try it and took me off Haldol. I was exhibiting gastrointestinal symptoms not normally associated with this type of drug and became dehydrated with extreme weight loss. After ten days in the hospital, it seemed the Haldol was finally out of my system and I began to improve.

Shivers encumber the child
Curled in the corner of a dark, cold room.
Bursts of wind flow freely about
Entering through the broken and shattered windows.
Pain and hunger
Thrust within the child's timid body
As he searches for a single morsel of food
Only to find himself too tired to move.
Sickness remains within him
As a cold goes long untreated.
Fear surrounds him
As he lies there throughout the night.
All hope is diminished
No one hears him cry
As he curls in the darkened corner.
He prays,
Hoping that his prayers will be answered
That he may be loved someday.

I spent ten days in the hospital. My mother came several times. She didn't say much, and I could see the pain and hurt in her eyes. My older sister stopped by with her church friends. They acted as if they were never going to see me again. I couldn't eat, and I could barely move. This didn't make things better. When I was finally able to go back to school, I looked like an anorexic. I remember walking the halls, alone. No one even knew I was gone. They never said a word. Then again, they never knew I was there. At home, it was the same. My brother and sister ignored me and my dad looked at me with what I felt was disgust. I felt abandoned; alone and afraid of the world that both surrounded me and kept me isolated.

I started on pimozide. It was quite similar to Haldol, only not as intense with the side effects. Since this was the last possible alternative known to us, I remained where I was.

Things were different this time around. Upon entering the ninth grade I had developed a slight speech problem that required therapy. Often I found myself repeating words or phrases that others have said. I wouldn't repeat it directly after, but would constantly incorporate it into my every day conversations. It often made people angry, as they mistook it for my making fun of them. I was often unaware of what they were accusing me.

> The rain is softly falling upon the leaves
> As I walk along the rivers edge.
> It is a quiet day.
> The birds are singing and fluttering about
> As the wind gently brushes through my hair.
> Slowly I walk
> Letting the water trickle between my toes.
> Farther down the path was a waterfall
> Excitement grew rapidly within me
> As I raced the rapids to reach it.
> While my heart quickened with my pace
> The water became violent.
> And the wind tugged harder at my hair
> The animals squealed and jumped about.
> The turbulent energy of that moment
> Filled my blood with anticipation.
> With one final plunge into the water
> The moment was gone.
> Once again the birds sang and fluttered about
> As the rapids again trickled slowly over the rocks
> And the wind gently blew in this world
> Where peace reigns
> Only to drown all violence and sorrow.

It all started like that. A simple thought of how the world would be without me. Death slowly became an obsession. All I could see was the turbulence and animosity that occurred wherever I went. No one cared for my company or opinion. They just wanted me out of their lives. I saw myself as a nuisance, disrupting others wherever I was. I closed out everything and everyone. Soon I found myself deeply depressed with no way out. The pain from home and school became too much to bear. Soon, it was the only thing I knew. In a way, it seemed to have befriended me, for it was always there. It was all I ever knew.

> Destruction of the soul
> Followed by a pain so deep
> A dagger cannot repeat its depth within the heart
> The darkness surrounds me
> Tugging at my fears
> And making them a dominant reality in the night.
> I am weakened by my own fear
> As my pain destroys me
> And my sorrow pulls at my heart relentlessly
> Until it shatters upon the floor
> Torn without mercy upon this Earth.
> The water flows above my head
> As my tears continue to drown me in my sorrow
> I cannot move
> As the life is drawn out from within me
> My soul now departed.
> The darkness has become my life;
> Pain, my only friend.

The depression had taken over my life. I walked, talked, and breathed death. It was all I thought about. Of course, I didn't let anyone know how I felt. I feared their rejection would only make it worse. I hid behind false smiles, and a laughter that was not mine. I never let anyone inside, and I never came out.

I started writing poetry my freshman year of High School. It usually contained pictures of painted fantasies. I used it to mask my true feelings while deep inside I was dead. I felt so dead that at times I even tried to make it reality. I overdosed several times. My failures only made me feel even worse, and more obsessed with ending my life. I thought it would bring peace to others, by not having to look at me.

Upon entering my sophomore year, I had started to express myself only through my poetry. The darkness often reflected upon the pain and isolation that filled my soul. The shadows were the hidden creatures that controlled my body (my Tourette syndrome). I always felt held back, denied the right to express what I felt. In my writing I spoke of light as if it were peace. Yet again, my obsessions with death set in. The only way I perceived peace to be possible was to end my life, thus securing the eternal light. This thought process only led to more attempted suicides and bouts of depression that seemed endless.

> I stand
> In the shadows of the night.
> As my fear grows strong
> The light
> It grows dim.
> As the fog draws closer
> Shutting out all hope of secureness
> I stand
> Searching for a light
> Any light
> To guide me to my home.
> But I am lost
> For I know not

Where my home is.
For the shadows of the night
Dance about my head
Twisting me
And pushing me down a spiral hole.
I sink
And I coil up
Locking all thoughts inside.
A light, glistens above me
Breaking the chain which holds me.
The fog slips away and I uncoil.
My thoughts becoming very dangerous
I tear at the night
Which blocks my vision.
I break free
The light now surrounds me
I am secure
I found my home
It is the eternal light.

December 27, 1987 marked a new beginning of sorts. It was the first day I stopped taking pimozide completely. A few months later, my depression began to subside. I had made a few friends who are still present today. I even had a boyfriend. Things at home, however, were still the same. I kept on writing poetry. I began to let people read it, often using it as a way of asking for help. I would never state it directly but would play with imagery or 'similar' situations to how I was feeling.

Laughing ...
A slight smile breaks upon your face
And you walk among your friends
Ignorant to the pains around you.

That man ...
He crouches in that corner ...
Cold ...
Hungry ...
And afraid
Each day passing, he begs you pay notice
To his needs.
To think you may feel compassion ...
Oh how wrong he was.
How can one feel compassion
For what one has not himself felt or needed.

Days go by
And your ignorance blocks all sight and pain
As you pass by the corner ...
Now empty.
But yet you notice not
For you have not felt the pains that lingered there.
As your life continues as before.

But I ...
I have seen his pains and felt them
I have given what life I could offer him
And in return gained respect for grief.
I have lived ...
Breathed and felt his pain
Until his dying day ...
Where I exist no more.

This was my way of asking for help, and that is exactly what I got. Mrs. Hoffman and Mrs. Berry, my reading and photography teachers, were my so called angels sent from heaven. In my writings and pictures they had noticed that something was wrong.

We talked often after school. They helped me deal with and overcome the depression that had become my life. They helped me realize that I wasn't a bad person. In order for others to accept me, I had to accept myself. This is where my new journey began.

Before, my relationships reflected upon my state of mind, as they were filled with anger and pain. I had convinced myself that it was love, for it was all I knew. I hated my life, and decided it was time for a change. I started to read the pamphlets my mother received from the Tourette Syndrome Association, and it was during this time that I realized what was wrong with me. I had trouble at first, but gradually began to accept the idea that I would have Tourette syndrome all my life. At times the thought is still too overwhelming. This change took place in my senior year at high school.

I looked upon college as a new beginning. It was a chance to erase my past while letting only a few select friends inside my mind to share my memories with. I began to discuss my Tourette syndrome among my close friends and the curious few who were courageous enough to ask about it. My tics had subsided a great deal, and talking about it brought great satisfaction. I did a report on Tourette syndrome for my biology class and not only did I receive a greater understanding, but also relief. I realized my other 'related problems' weren't me, but were the Tourette syndrome acting inside me. I realized the source behind my constant desire for death, and eventually enlightenment came. The summer following my freshman year, I participated in a SPECT (Single Photon Emission Computerized Tomography) study. I went there in the hope of not only learning more about Tourette syndrome, but to meet others who had it as well. I realized that I felt so alone. My friends and family had no idea what it was like to be me; to crouch in pain as others ridiculed you. I thought that by meeting someone else with Tourette syndrome, I would no longer feel so alone.

I met a fellow patient there named John. At first I was very hesitant to open up, only because he was 'ticing' so freely. I wasn't ashamed of him. Without realizing it, I thought he was mocking me like everyone else. But then I remembered he has Tourette syndrome, and that was just him. We talked for hours about our past and our struggles with Tourette syndrome. It felt good knowing that I could just be myself, that someone else understood what I was going through. I realized I am not alone. John had helped me accept it for what it is, and to love me for whom I am. No one can change that.

> The shadows were closing in on me.
> Yet I walked on,
> Deep into the woods.
> My fears were no longer mine
> For I had given them up days ago.
> My pains ...
> Now only memories to be reflected upon
> And learned from in the days to come.
> I walk freely within the woods
> Feeling the life that surrounds me
> And living the emotions that fill my soul.
> Deepened by the pleasures of the woods,
> I smile ...
> Carefree and at peace.
> No harm to me can come
> In this sacred world
> Of strange and new desires
> With which I live.
> I scope the land
> Like a sacred bird,
> And I am truly free.
> I AM ME ... Forever.

Realizing who I am has made life more bearable. My tics are gradually becoming worse again, as they affect my wrists and fingers, and eyes. Sometimes I would have bouts of multiple tics resembling seizures. This new understanding has made it more tolerable. I have even found that by taking an aspirin, and pretending to have overdosed, it would alleviate the urge to die. This has brought great relief upon me as well as my friends. I have even decided to join the Tourette Syndrome Association support group, so that I can share my experiences and learn even more about it. Most important, that I may know I'm not alone in this fight. Someday I hope to conduct research on Tourette syndrome in the effort toward finding its cause and a cure.

Looking back, many things have happened in my life, most of them painful. Sometimes, even the memory of things brings tears to my eyes. I realize now that I was never alone. Without the strength and love of Jesus, I wouldn't be alive today.

> I have reached a point in my life
> Where nothing matters.
> My thoughts are carefree
> And my actions speak for words.
> No longer do I have to worry
> About past memories or pains.
> No longer do I dwell
> On what is to come.
> I live for now,
> And now is the moment in time
> When my life is forever long and beautiful.
> My guides are angelic in nature
> And they see me through hard times.
> I cannot see or feel pain,
> Yet I know its presence
> And I understand.

I live for you,
As you have given me a life to live.
I know you . . .
I love you . . .
And you are there for me always.
Your love is never ending.

A BETTER PERSON WITH TOURETTE SYNDROME

by

Matt Foulkrod
as told to John S. Hilkevich

In my first course as a graduate student in Counseling Services, my professor mentioned the uniqueness of establishing a rapport with a Tourette syndrome client of his. My professor spoke anonymously of the client, a twelve year old boy with socialization problems. During a class break, I pulled the professor aside and quietly told him that I knew something about Tourette syndrome; that I suffered from it. That was the first time, other than a casual passing mention, I spoke to anyone about my Tourette syndrome. This was before I met anyone with Tourette syndrome, before "official" medical diagnosis, before viewing the Tourette Syndrome Association videos. Looking back, I am

*amazed at how difficult it was to share my Tourette syndrome
with this professor. With Matt's parents' permission, he referred
me to them as a resource. Matt marked my first "Tourette
syndrome referral" and out of that a friendship grew between his
family and me. His contribution to this book strikes a note of
fondness in me and an anchor to my own story of coming out
about Tourette syndrome.*

*Soon after our first meeting, Matt, his father, my father, my
brother-in-law, and a small group of Tourette syndrome affected
children and their parents rappelled down into a "wild" (non-
commercial) cave. Upon exiting the abyss where there is no light,
no weather, no change, and waiting for others to climb out, I
heard Matt quizzing the other children on the nature of their
Tourette syndrome. As I was belaying the remaining cavers on
their climb out, a thought kept slamming at me: "What if I, at age
twelve, could have done what Matt is doing now, where and who
would I be today in my growth?" Irony also struck me: I am three
times older than Matt, and yet he, in one important way, is ahead
of me. That is why I wanted him to have his say, and why I want
to continue to watch his story unfold.*

John S. Hilkevich

It was in the first grade when I started noticing things were
different about me from the other kids. Things that were, to say
the least, weird . . . I rolled my eyes, made strange faces at the
teacher who took it personally, and found myself barking and
sniffing and clearing my throat. At summer camp that year my
arm flapping earned me the name of "Chicken Man." I began
getting mad at the whole world and confused about what was
going on in me.

Second grade made IT worse. I was different and bigger

than the other kids and constantly picked on, picking fights, calling me names. When I was in little league baseball, I was just an average player and the other kids on the team hassled me, kids who had similar behavior problems as me, maybe worse! The second grade teacher treated everybody in the class the same no matter how smart or stupid or different they were. I was always in the girls' reading group because I was one of the better readers, but I was angry because I still wanted to be with the people I hung around with. It was a bad year due to the misunderstanding of the teachers and students of my condition.

I was always getting blamed for things I didn't do. Once a girl found a note in her little mailbox that said "I hate you!" It wasn't in my handwriting but I still got blamed. I was constantly having to write these sentences, "I will not do this or that, etc," and being singled out and set up by my classmates because I wasn't liked and they were afraid of me and my strangeness.

Fourth grade was a great break for me. I was still playing baseball and having fun and was one of the better students in my classes. I still didn't know what I had, and I was still scared. But because my teacher helped, understood and listened to me, I really enjoyed that year.

Fifth grade was utter hell. The beatings from the other kids got worse and I came home with bruises. Besides the weird things I already mentioned, my compulsions to touch things in a certain way, to walk on certain tiles a certain amount of times in my kitchen, to walk in a ridiculous way, staring at things for a certain amount of time, scraping every crumb off my plates, touching and tapping people in the arms and shoulders . . . things that I had to do or my body would fill with an unbelievable tension . . . got worse and expanded in number.

The obsessive-compulsiveness sometimes led to people getting hurt physically and emotionally, and serious disciplinary actions, although I wasn't always at fault. I felt unfairly treated, often a scapegoat. Sometimes I liked myself and other times life wasn't worth living because I couldn't accomplish what I wanted. I felt like dying at times. People don't understand that Tourette syndrome runs deeper than making noises and movements . . . it involves such feelings as abuse and inner hatred and emotional pain that encourages fantasies of suicide and death.

Concerns of my doctor and parents grew to the point where a battery of tests were ordered, such as psychological interviews, EEGs, MRIs, blood work, balance tests and other neurological evaluations. After three months of testing, I was finally diagnosed with Tourette syndrome. I was ecstatic and relieved that all the things I was doing had a name and a reason. It got better at school now that I knew what I had and was better understood and accepted. Soon after that I went to a Christian day camp that I loved and changed my life. The medications that were prescribed for me helped to make daily living easier, but not without side effects such as gaining a lot of weight. School still presented its problems, (one reading teacher would send me out of the room for making noises) and they wanted to classify me as SED (severely emotionally disturbed). One teacher helped to fight that label since it wasn't me. I have Tourette syndrome. My grades, though, were getting worse and I became frequently interested in just having fun as the school work got harder. My parents looked into getting me into a private school and I was given another battery of tests and given the label ADD (attention deficit disorder). I did get accepted in a private school that I love and I'm getting good grades. And I've gotten used to Tourette syndrome . . . It's just the way I am.

I do plan to go to college, not only to make my parents happy, but also to make me feel better about myself and to get a good job. I want to major in biology and geology to learn more about nature as I want to work in the outdoors. Learning about and doing search and rescue work would be part of that, making me feel even better about myself by helping others. That's good therapy for Tourette syndrome persons.

Marriage is another goal in my life. Any woman going out with or marrying someone with Tourette syndrome needs to be very understanding. I would be looking very early for Tourette syndrome symptoms in my kids and would hope they wouldn't have it. People with Tourette syndrome are better able to detect it in kids because we know and understand symptoms that others would not even notice. I, having grown up with Tourette syndrome, would be more understanding with my kid's behaviors and tics and their needs, such as extra opportunities to socialize.

Nobody should pick on others for the fun of it. Tourette syndrome people especially know what it's like to be harassed and tend to be more respectful of other's feelings. People with Tourette syndrome need to work extra hard and I encourage them to strive for their utmost potential.

Given the chance not to have Tourette syndrome I would decline, it is part of myself. Sometimes I wonder that if I didn't have Tourette syndrome, would I be who I am now? I feel that Tourette syndrome has made me a better person and I would not want to be anyone else.

JUST AN ORDINARY KID

by

Kevin R. Pratt
as told to Lindy Thomas

By the time this book is in its first printing, Kevin will be fifteen years old. He, Matt and the other youthful contributors are of the first generation that Adam points out in his <u>In the Group</u> chapter, as the beneficiaries of more speedy and accurate diagnosis . . . the long lapses before a correct diagnosis , the years of confusion, pain and struggles will gratefully end with my generation, largely to the credit of the Tourette Syndrome Association Kevin's family is part of that gift to the Tourette syndrome community. His mother is the director of the South Jersey Tourette Syndrome Association chapter. It was his family that embraced my entrance into the Tourette syndrome world of support, understanding and love. I am tearfully grateful to them.
Early diagnosis or not, Kevin amazes me . . . with his

compassionate sensitivity to others with various handicaps, with his demonstrative and uninhibited giving of affection to his younger siblings, with his healthy and rich socialization, (he has many good friends of both genders,) with his stable and appropriate public and school conduct, with his athletic and academic progress and achievements. On our Tourette Syndrome Chapter's first adventure workshop (cliff rappelling and climbing) Kevin wore a T shirt with the inscription, "Tourette syndrome; Ask me about it." During his school's science fair, he stood by his project, a display on Tourette syndrome, inviting people to "ask me about it." He, like Matt and the other Tourette syndrome teens, would have been role models for me when I was 15. They, unborn in my youth, now enter my life as teachers for me. Where do they get their self-acceptance, their courage to be vulnerable in opening their lives in their neighborhoods and to the world in this book? And Kevin calls himself, "Just an Ordinary Kid." I know what you mean, Kevin, but you're not "just...," you're a very special ordinary kid.

John S. Hilkevich

This is the hardest thing I have ever had to do in my life. . . to write about it! I don't really even want to think about IT, let alone write about IT for all the world to see. I have always felt that IT was my own private problem. That is probably why I never got really angry when someone stared at me or made fun of me on the playground. BUT . . . they told me that my story might help other kids who have Tourette syndrome like me and that is why I decided to do it.

My name is Kevin. At the time I am writing this, I am fourteen years old. I have a mom, two dads, two brothers and sisters. I am the second oldest kid in the family. I love playing soccer and riding around town on my bike. I like to visit my grandmother's house and see my cousins. My favorite hockey team is the Los Angeles Kings and my favorite food is pizza. I used to collect California Raisins, but I don't do kid stuff like that anymore. Now I collect coins and go to a vocational high school. I want to be a cook when I graduate.

My best friend is Roger. I'm going to talk a lot about Roger in this story because he has been my friend for a long time. He was with me before I had IT, and he was with me right after I found out what IT was, and he is still with me now. And something else that Roger always did was stick up for me. When the going would get a little rough on the playground, Roger was always there. Sometimes he would tell them to leave me alone, sometimes he and I would just walk away. But it is a lot easier to walk away when you have someone to walk away with. I guess besides my family, he is the most important person in my life.

When I was little, IT hadn't shown up yet. I remember silly stuff. Like sleeping in a room with my brother, Steven. Like the airplane that hung over my bed. Like being afraid of the dark. And I remember sitting on my mother's lap. Once I went out in the street. I can still see and hear my dad saying "NO NO!" My mom tells everyone that I was very kind to people who had handicaps — like this little girl I knew in a wheelchair. She seems to think that deep inside I knew even then about that sort of thing. But I don't know, you know how mothers are.

In kindergarten, I was just like everyone else. I learned that the door was on the left and that the windows were on the right. I learned my alphabet. Roger and I rode our BIG WHEELS together and we ate dinner at each other's houses.

In first grade there was an eclipse. I remember closing my eyes and not looking at it for fear of becoming blind. (It's funny how afraid of stuff you are when you are a little kid.) I also learned how to tell time in first grade and I got my first watch.

Yes, I'd say I started out to have a pretty normal life. In fact, IT never showed up until I was in second grade. At first, they thought it was a speech problem, (because I made funny sounds in my throat.) I also started shaking my head and blinking my eyes a lot. When the other kids told me to stop I got really mad. The teacher also kept sending me to the nurse to have my ears and eyes checked. Often I just wanted to go home. I wasn't enjoying school anymore at all. Most of the time all this put me in a really bad mood. Sometimes I would fight with my brother or tease my sister until I made her cry. Then that would make my mom and pop mad at me. I can't really blame them. It's just that I was so miserable myself I couldn't be nice to anyone else.

Third grade wasn't any better. Actually things got much worse. One day my math teacher even took me out in the hall to ask me if I wanted to take off my outside shirt. She thought I must be hot if I was shaking that much. That was pretty embarrassing. It was also embarrassing when a girl who was usually nice to me, looked me right in the eye and asked, "Why do you shake your head?" Of course, since IT didn't have a name yet, I had to answer, "I don't know." Boy, talk about wanting to disappear. But I couldn't disappear, I just had to go on day after day shaking and blinking.

After school I got to be with Roger and my buddies. In our gang everyone got made fun for one reason or another. Two guys were kind of ... well ... chunky and one kid looked Japanese. So it wasn't too bad getting made fun of if everybody else was too. We did kid stuff like wrestle and play video games. There was this one video game that we played that always got me teased more than anyone else. It was called "Chuck Norris" and it made this sound like ... "VVVVT." Well every time Chuck went "VVVVT," I would make a sound like "HUT HUT." That would really get on everyone's nerves after a while. You better believe I got so I hated to play that game.

Then came fourth grade and I kind of black out. My teacher says that I got under a desk and barked like a dog. I honestly cannot remember doing that. I'm not saying that she is lying or anything. Its just that I can't remember it. My sister says that kids were asking her about me in the bathroom what was wrong with me. Of course she didn't know what to say. Nobody knew what IT was . . . I guess when something bad happens to you, sometimes your mind just doesn't want to think about it. Some things I do remember though . . . like being afraid that I might die, and wondering what was going to happen to me when I grew up. I also remember asking God to make IT go away. In church while the minister said his prayers for the sick people, I asked God to take IT away. I know that my mom and everyone was really worried about me. Mom tried everything to help me but nothing seemed to work. Everyone kept trying to give my mom advice they thought would help me. They told her not to make a big deal out of it because it would just make it worse. They said it could be an emotional problem since my mom and dad had gotten a divorce and all. I knew it wasn't that, but who listens to a little kid?

Anyway . . . that was the year that my mom read the article in Ann Landers. It described a kid just like me. Then she took me to the doctor. He said, "I think you have hit the nail right on the head." Next we went to the hospital. They told mom about a support group that led us right into the arms of my wonderful doctor. He is still my doctor today. He knew ALL about IT, and how to help me, and how to help mom too. Mom says it was a miracle that we found him. Maybe he was the answer to all those prayers I had prayed in church. Who knows?

Sure enough IT had a name: Tourette syndrome, named after the guy who discovered it. Well that was the best and the worst day of my life. I found out that I wasn't going to die. That was good. But I also found out that it wasn't going to go away. There was no cure for it. Also I found out that it might get worse as I grew up. When I got home, guess what I did? I went right to Roger. I told him everything. He listened to the whole thing and said he was sorry. I found out later that he told the rest of the gang. It was weird what happened. Not only did the guys stop cutting on me, they stopped teasing everyone! They asked me some questions like, "Are you unconscious when you twitch?" At least they were questions that I could answer. You couldn't blame them for being curious. After all I was the only person that they knew with Tourette syndrome.

Meanwhile my mom got real busy. Now she was able to do all sorts of things to help me. She called the school and had a talk with all of my teachers. By the time I started fifth grade they knew about my disease. The teacher helped the kids in my class to know more about Tourette syndrome. That really helped with the questions and the teasing. My mom also got me a tutor to help me with my school work and to help me get my papers organized. (We never did decide if that was the Tourette syndrome or just me.) But my mom got me the help anyway. My mom also found out that there is a medicine that I could take to help the ticcing. It is called Haldol. At first it made me real sleepy, but now it doesn't really bother me that much. Until they got the medicine regulated, I fell asleep in school a lot. I also got bad headaches. Sometimes I had to come home in the middle of the day.

In seventh and eighth grade I went to a special class for extra help. I got to take my tests without being timed. The doctor said that I should have that so my mom made sure the school gave it to me. Most of the teachers were really understanding. So was the nurse. One of my teachers (when she noticed that I was having a bad day) would get me to tell her EMOTIONAL or PHYSICAL. If it were emotional we would either talk about it or I could write about it in my journal. My mom and I joined a support group so that we could get to know other people who have Tourette syndrome. I like going to the meetings. The kids talk to each other while the adults talk to each other. We help each other.

In a way I think I am really lucky. There are many people who have Tourette syndrome a lot worse than I do. I feel sorry for them, but I am glad that I don't have it really bad. Another thing I never did that other people do is try to stop a tic. The medicine tries to stop them, but I never did. Maybe that is why I never got as nervous as other people. But then I have to remember that maybe my tics aren't as bad as theirs. This November my mom is taking me to the Tourette Syndrome Association National Convention. I can't wait! I get to stay in a hotel and see how a real cook does his job. I'm sure that I will meet people worse and better off than me.

I'm not trying to say that finding out made my life into the perfect life or anything. I still get into my share of trouble — at home and at school too. (And I would be in trouble right now if my mom found out that last week Roger and I "nuked" a frog in a microwave.) I still like to tease my sister, Karen. I still get into fights with my brothers, Steven and Charlie. (Oh, I forgot to tell you. We have a new kid in the family. Baby Ashley is nine months old. Now she is really something! I love making funny faces at her and seeing her laugh.) But I do want to say that finding out that you have a disease is better than not knowing what you have. The more you find out about it, the less scared you are. And even if people ask you what is wrong, it's easier to say "I have Tourette syndrome" than to have to say "I don't know." By the time I got into eighth grade, I even did my Science Project on Tourette syndrome. Tourette syndrome will always be a part of my life, but it is not *running* or *ruining* my life anymore.

Finally, for anyone who reads this story, there are some things I want to tell you:

1. Be yourself, you are OK inside, even if the outside shakes.

2. Go with your life. Have goals and work toward them. You can do anything that you want to do.

3. There are people who will be your friend. Keep looking if you haven't found one yet.

4. If you think that God isn't listening to you, He is. He just really wants you to love yourself anyway. Remember . . . nobody's perfect.

I am Kevin's mom. He wrote how much easier it was to walk away from a negative challenge when someone walked with him. Let me tell you how it was easier for me to walk into a challenge when someone special walked with me. That was Lindy, who helped Kevin put his story down to paper: she walked with me through doctor's appointments; through group support meetings; through the tightly closed doors of child study teams and the educational bureaucracy. Thank you, Lindy, for your sacrifice, patience, understanding and love . . . most of all, for helping my son and me walk the journey that led to whom he is today. I love you.

Debbie

PURPOSE

by

Wayne Martin

I met Wayne Martin in Medford, Oregon, while on tour speaking to Tourette Syndrome Association chapters throughout the fall of 1991. At dinner the night before the two of us seemed in competition to drink the most water and joked about our liquid needs. Wayne had never been an alcoholic but in his profession worked with them and offered me some much needed advice on the problems I was facing in early sobriety.

The issue of employment discrimination is an important one to adults with Tourette syndrome, but there is little in the literature about this problem. Wayne eloquently addresses this in his contribution to our book.

Adam Ward Seligman

Wayne Martin

Purpose, something to do that is meaningful. Purpose is a cure for failure. Al Bundy, the fictional shoe salesman on *Married With Children* claims his life has no purpose, yet people do need shoes. Perhaps purpose is like Tourette syndrome. Just as one's purpose in life varies from person to person, so do the symptoms of Tourette syndrome. As Touretters, we often question this sometimes baffling, always annoying malady that plagues our lives. That we choose to fight back, refusing to be conquered by Tourette syndrome, gives our lives value. If I choose to, I could simply say that I have an illness and there is nothing I can do about it. A more accurate statement, however, would be that I have an illness and I choose to do nothing about it. By making the conscious choice to change or at least attempt to control Tourette syndrome rather than allowing Tourette syndrome to control us, we have established a purpose in our lives. By accepting this simple reasoning, we are forced to admit that our life has purpose, and with that purpose, comes meaning, and with meaning self-esteem and the respect of our peers. But, without purpose, we will wallow in the Al Bundy mentality, sinking ever so slowly into the abyss.

Putting into words what Tourette syndrome has meant to my life took some thinking. After running various scenarios through my mind, looking for good catch words, trying to find that sentence or sentences that sum up my feelings, it came to me. It was so simple. How has Tourette syndrome affected my life? It has given me purpose. But it wasn't always so.

To me Tourette syndrome is a relatively new phrase in my life. Five years ago I could not have told you what it was, let alone discussed it. Today I quote the experts as I attempt to educate the ignorant, remembering that just five short years ago I too was ignorant. They say that ignorance is bliss. I say ignorance is pain, and in my case it is a pain that I deal with everyday.

My earliest remembrances of Tourette syndrome go back to

the age of five. I am sure there were symptoms before age five, but I find as I grow older that memories that once readily jumped out of my mind have now drifted away and become part of an unremembered past. At age five, I started school. My phobia of school began on day one and I don't believe it has ever really left. To this day the smell of new school clothes gives me butterflies. It's funny the things you remember after forty-three years of life. I remember going to the doctor because I was always stomping on my toes. I could not explain why and, worse yet, neither could the doctor. Tourette syndrome, I now realize, was the culprit. The realization hurts as I look at broken, twisted toes.

I remember the need to be always getting a drink of water. To this day I recall the cool refreshing drink one could get by the meat counter at Hagestrom's Grocery. The store has been gone a good thirty years, yet the memory is there. Today I can tell you where every drinking fountain is in every store I've been in. Dr. David Comings provided the answer to my questions about my need to consume and my fascination with water. It is called polydipsia.

I remember the embarrassment, sitting in a junior high school counselor's office receiving my scores on achievement tests. He wondered if I had been ill that day. In retrospect, I guess he was right. I remember machine shop in high school and the teacher's admonition that if you weren't careful you could end up a broken mass if the machine got you. Stephen King could not have put more fear into me. I flunked the first quarter. My projects were a mess but I was always on time.

In college, the mind that could not master introduction to algebra or whether a word ended in s' or 's was able to memorize fifty-two pages of handwritten notes, verbatim, in a week's time.

The adult who now feels the urge to wash his hands each time he shakes someone's hand is the same person whom as a child always washed his toy cars before putting them away after play.

From an adult point of view, the worst thing I have dealt with as a Touretter has been discrimination in the work place. I spent the first five and half years out of high school working in a service station. I was good but I did not get promotions. For many months I was the top salesperson. I stood back as others moved forward and my anger built. I looked for other jobs but couldn't find any. Each rejection was a setback. I finally just quit, and walked away, hurt, and angry.

A few months later I went to work as a sprinkler setter for a school district. This was a night job. I worked by myself. Not a good place for someone who is afraid of dark places. From there I went on to be a custodian in a junior high school. I worked hard and did my job. The boss was always on me. I think it was because he was full of crap and he knew that I knew it.

A move to Oregon in 1973 set a new course for my life. I worked again as a janitor but only until I got residency in the state and could go to school. In college, I excelled. I began to think of myself as an 'A' student and mentally berated myself if I got a lesser grade. I also realized that many professors saw me as an 'A' student. I did good work. I was a methodical student. I had entered college with forty transfer credits. Twenty-seven months later I left with two bachelor degrees and within a year of graduation completed an additional forty-five credits needed for a master's degree. This was followed by ten months of unemployment. I quit saving rejection slips when I got to fifty-three. It took twenty-three interviews to get a job. I was even turned down by people with whom I had gone to college. The thought of an interview sent terror through me. It still does. After a sleepless night, I would awake with a nervous stomach. I would arrive twenty to thirty minutes before the interview. That time was spent massaging my toes and mentally praying that I could keep my feet still during the interview. I learned quickly to let my neck tic only when the interviewers looked down at their papers. I also had the occasional lapse in memory and was mortified when I had to stop in mid response to ask what the question was.

My first post college job was a CETA placement in a counseling office for $700.00 per month. My boss who wrote me a letter of recommendation when leaving would later tell me privately that she would not have hired me back. That hurt. It still does. Other jobs followed and I returned to college as a part time student to complete an additional bachelor's degree as well as a teaching credential. My total college grade point average was 3.5 on a 4.0 scale. I am very proud of this.

I have always been an advocate of the underdog and always rooted for those seeking change, always stood behind those who refused to be corrupted. My first job after college, this time, ended fifteen months later. I chose to stand up for my beliefs. I was fired and spent the next two years in and out of court and in and out of private counseling sessions. I saw two medical doctors, who said I was under stress. I saw a Ph.D., who said I was faking my symptoms. I saw a Ph.D., who didn't want to be involved in a worker's compensation claim. Lastly I saw another Ph.D., who listened and was compassionate. None of these professionals recognized the symptoms of Tourette syndrome that were outwardly very visible.

The best I could do job wise for the next four years was to work as a substitute school teacher. When I did not get a job, I asked why. After asking why a few times, I quit getting interviews. I also worked part time for a community college teaching adult education. It was my boss at the college who first handed me the blue pamphlet from the National Tourette Syndrome Association. At the time I was still seeing the compassionate Ph.D. who listened. When I told him I thought I might have Tourette syndrome, he said he thought I might be right. When, after talking further, he realized that I was a Touretter, he apologized for

missing the symptoms. My personal reaction was one of profound relief. At last I had some answers. I was thirty eight years
old. Within two years, my boss at the college, the 'enlightened
person' who had realized I had Tourette syndrome had let me go
with no explanation and no chance of rehire. That still hurts.
About six months of unemployment followed. Discrimination is
demoralizing and it hurts. Like the African American who is
discriminated against because of his color, the Tourette American is discriminated against because of his outward symptoms.
Neither of us can change but we can work to change the way
people treat us.

That brings us to today, where you will find me working as
a Substance Abuse Counselor. Until recently I worked for two
bosses who professed to understand Tourette syndrome. They
did not! I was the best educated employee they had and yet I was
one of the lowest paid. Why? I am angry. I am hurt. I fight back
but the discrimination continues.

As a Substance Abuse Counselor I have an opportunity to
help other people with Tourette syndrome, for those who have
Tourette syndrome show up in great numbers in chemical depen-
dency programs. In three years I have identified approximately
twenty men and women with Tourette syndrome. They have, for
the most part, been alcoholic. They have been through a criminal
justice system that looks only at the facts. Judges, attorneys and
the police often have no idea what Tourette syndrome is. All they
know is that they are dealing with an addict or a drunk driver. To
make matters worse, many social workers remain ignorant of
Tourette syndrome and its manifestations. To me, at this point
discrimination becomes synonymous with misdiagnosis. I have
seen clients who are clearly suffering from Tourette syndrome,
mistreated, mismedicated and returned to court because of non
compliance. The treatment community must open its eyes and its
minds. Asking the right questions, taking a good family history,

and looking at past criminal activity can help to identify a person with Tourette syndrome. Misdiagnosis is discrimination and ignorance is not an excuse.

Outside of the treatment community it is up to people with Tourette syndrome to educate. Discrimination is rampant. We must be heard by the school systems, written about in the media and understood by employers. I know we can make a difference.

Frank Sinatra says "I did it my way." I guess that sums up my life. To those who have hurt me, I will tell you I will never forget. To those who have helped-me, I say thank you. As my fellow Touretters will tell you, we never forget an argument or a slight just as we never forget a helping hand. Together we shall educate. Discrimination against Touretters will end. The future will be brighter for youngsters with Tourette syndrome, for myself and other adults are out there teaching people that Tourette syndrome can be dealt with and those who have it can live a normal life and get the jobs for which they are qualified. As adults and children alike with Tourette syndrome, we have a purpose. I have a purpose.

THREE AT A TIME

by

Rose Wood

The knowledge that Tourette syndrome is genetic was always a great relief to me. It seemed to confirm that the disorder was physical, not psychological. It also allowed me to understand and even to forgive my grandfather his rages and outbursts that were so often directed at my grandmother. While my grandfather was never diagnosed, we did have a misdiagnosis from 1911 of St. Vitus Dance, now known as Sydenham's Chorea, another movement disorder. Sydenham's Chorea didn't include vocal tics and these my grandfather most definitely had.

The genetic aspects of Tourette syndrome were reassuring to me. To others the gene resulted in tragedy. In Rose Wood's story, and the two that follow, what shows up in multiple cases of Tourette syndrome created tension in the family almost destroying it. But through her strength, Rose survived three cases of Tourette syndrome.

Rose is active in the Metropolitan Detroit Tourette Syndrome Association, and is starting her own business as a mediator in parent - school conflicts involving children with Tourette syndrome, Attention Deficit Disorder and Learning Disabilities. Currently she works as a social worker. She is writing a book for children about Tourette syndrome.

Adam Ward Seligman

I am a wife and a mother of Touretters.

Prior to marriage my husband made a low sounding growl, a sound I took as a sign of his affection for me. He also had a cute little twitch that I would tease him about. Since the age of 12, Larry was a heavy coffee drinker (stimulant) and a heavy smoker (nicotine has been known to minimize tics.)

When our son Andrew, was diagnosed with asthma, Larry went on a health kick and stopped smoking and drinking coffee. Shortly after, he developed mood swings, outbursts, was seemingly more disorganized and unable to complete tasks. When he was driving a car or resting, he developed head, shoulder, and arm, motor tics. When resting or relaxing, the growl was more prominent. He began to experience eye problems and his inability to focus was a concern. He saw an opthalmologist who diagnosed nystagmus as the culprit.

He was becoming a changed man. I thought he had a brain tumor and suggested he see a neurologist. After a battery of tests, we were informed that he had tics, nervous habits. Should they become worse or should he loose consciousness, then we were instructed to request medication to help him.

During this time, Andrew was two and a half and began to mimic his father. He was corrected and told "Dad can't help what he does. Stop It!" Andrew began to make noises at preschool. He and his Dad were becoming the best of friends and the worst of enemies. They began to trigger each other and if I tried to intervene we would have a three ring scenario and this would intensify their outbursts.

Andrew would make annoying sounds at church like percussive hiccoughs, and other anti-social sounds. He was warned to stop and given consequences for his rude behavior, yet he'd continue making noises. I started to dislike my family. Andrew was a stubborn, resistant little brat. My husband was an inappropriate, out of control adult whose behaviors were sabotaging my disciplinary actions, with Andrew, and negating him as an appropriate role model for our son. My relationship with them became very strained.

From ages 3 to 6, Andrew was displaying many behavioral problems. For a child who was reading at 10 months old and operating a computer at 18 months old, none of his preschool work was being completed and he refused to participate in any coloring or any written activity. He was sassing, having problems with his peers, being impulsive, unpredictable and very difficult to manage. He was considered a class clown. He was manipulative, oppositional and continued to become unbearable. I was feeling less in control, frustrated and I felt I must be a bad wife and mother.

Because Andrew was so intelligent one psychologist diagnosed him as suffering from "infantile omnipresence."

Another psychologist said he was gifted in some areas but he had a significant gap between his performance IQ and his non-performance IQ. A third psychologist wanted to institutionalize Andrew to control the disorder. A fourth psychologist wanted me to divorce my husband and put Andrew in a public school ... that would fix everything. A fifth psychologist diagnosed Andrew and Larry with ADHD (Attention Deficit Hyperactivity Disorder).

The family therapist wasn't sure what was going on but agreed ADHD symptoms certainly matched my complaints of inattentiveness, distractibility, poor impulse control, and frustrations. We were referred back to our pediatrician and to a psychiatrist.

Andrew was started on Ritalin and within a week he had developed severe eye and facial tics. Ritalin was discontinued. The psychiatrist ordered another medication and Andrew developed another adverse reaction.

A teacher in my son's school came to me explaining that Andrew may have Tourette syndrome. Was she speaking a foreign language or what? Another person from the ADHD Support Group also suggested Tourette syndrome as a possible factor. I took Andrew to a neurologist who confirmed the diagnosis after taking a family history and performing tests to rule out other maladies. Later Emily, age four, was sniffing and making throat noises while relaxing in front of the T.V. She would cry, "Mommy, make it stop!" Having her diagnosed was not easy. They said she had "learned behavior" or was mimicing her brother. Eventually Emily was also diagnosed. Andrew and Emily were started on clonidine combined with the Ritalin and we finally had some positive results.

Larry could accept the diagnosis of ADHD but there wasn't any way he was going to accept the diagnosis of

Tourette syndrome. This became an issue which would later threaten our marriage.

A year later, as Andrew's asthma required more medication, his Tourette syndrome waxed and waned. The neurologist felt Andrew was too complicated and referred us to another neurologist. The second neurologist hospitalized Andrew long enough to wean Andrew off medication. A two day hospitalization is hardly long enough for clonidine to exit the system. Despite staff documentation of outbursts and tics, Andrew was released home. This action fed into my husband's denial. I was to try Andrew off medication or else...

At a public school Andrew was able to attend, the district hired a one-on-one aide and despite her help and mine, Andrew was still out of control. His behaviors were excessive and non-responsive to positive or negative discipline. He was unable to suppress anti-social behaviors and verbiage.

We were in crisis. I was near a nervous breakdown and a divorce. I was being accused of wanting the world on medication. I was a bad mother who didn't know how to discipline my children. I was rejected by my husband and my family members who believed Larry.

To them I was obsessed with this and was shoving it down their throats. What they didn't realize was I was fighting for my children and their futures, their self esteem. I wasn't as obsessed with it as it was devouring me. I would look forward to a quiet moment at home when the phone would ring for me to come over to the school.

Finally I decided that even if I had to divorce Larry, this had to stop. It was abusive to expect a child to discontinue behavior he could not control. I gave my husband an ultimatum to meet us at the psychiatrist or stay at work. I said we were going whether he came or not.

The psychiatrist realized that it was necessary to hospitalize Andrew. I think she just had to look at me to know she would hospitalize Andrew or she'd have to hospitalize me. The sad addition is Andrew wanted to be hospitalized. He wanted his medication. He knew he was out of control and was pleading for help. He "hated" and to this day "hates" the neurologist who took him off the medication in the first place.

The diagnosis was confirmed. He had ADHD and Tourette syndrome. He also had a learning disability and the associated behaviors related to Tourette syndrome; the inability to suppress angry thoughts, words or behaviors. Andrew was medicated. After a month of hospitalization, he returned to school to eventually no longer needing me or the aide. My husband reluctantly began to accept Tourette syndrome.

It is difficult living in a family where three members have Tourette syndrome and the associated behaviors (especially as we near medication time or early morning.) Life is definitely a challenge and unpredictable. I've learned much about life, human behavior and patience. I now am not as ready to look at a child or his caretakers as "bad."

My three Touretters are very intelligent and creative people who have a wonderful sense of humor. I think it helps them cope. I'm not a bad mother. Actually I'm one of the best.

THE FAMILY TOURETTE

by

Richard Stickann

In Rose Wood's story we saw how a non-affected parent dealt with Tourette syndrome. In Richard Stickann's story we see how a man with Tourette syndrome deals with having three children with the disorder. This chapter has one of the most engrossing descriptions of Obsessive Compulsive Disorder I have ever read.

Richard is a historian and writes for Western magazines. This is his first piece about Tourette syndrome.

Adam Ward Seligman

Richard Stickann

Tourette syndrome is a neurological disorder manifested by involuntary motor and vocal tics. There is no telethon raising money to find cures; the media pays little attention to it; it is a term that is not readily identifiable to most of the population. What dramatizations have been presented on TV have been misleading because Tourette syndrome is multi-dimensional carrying with it so many unpredictable and uncontrollable symptoms that are only the starting point leading to frustration, discouragement and distress.

Despite how debilitating Tourette syndrome might be on its victims, there is a positive side to the condition usually revealed through perserverence. Both the positive and negative elements of Tourette syndrome will be presented in this story.

This is a true account of a family that has been burdened with Tourette syndrome. It is a real family, in many ways like most other families.

It is a story about attitudes: five victims of Tourette syndrome all with different symptoms, different elements and how they are fighting to cope with this affliction and how as a family they have been burdened with the task of accepting Tourette syndrome as part of their lives and are trying to get on with the business of living those lives.

The Father
It is like a dark, murky night that never ends; relief is brief and superficial, and then abruptly consumed. There is a sense of hopelessness that what his body feels is constant. The sensations are real, sometimes obscure, often frightening, never absent.

His body experiences a continuing series of peaks and valleys, but where, in other circumstances, the peak may mean elation or ecstasy and the valley tranquility, for the father the peak brings strain, confusion and pain, a sense that an unseen, unknown and unwelcome pressure is poking, pushing and shoving every part of his body.

It is closing doors time and time again until sensations inside him announce "It is okay now, the door is closed correctly," even though he knew it was closed correctly the first, second, third time and every time after that. It was closed correctly even when the muscles in his hand and wrist contort in pain from grasping the door handle so many times until it is the "correct" time.

It is rolling up the car window a dozen times, locking doors over and over again, wringing out wet rags to the point where every muscle and bone in his hand aches. It is turning lights on and off dozens of times until he has halved the life expectancy of the bulb.

It is reading a sentence in a book or in a newspaper four, five, six or so many times that he has memorized it. But it must be done correctly, eyes beginning on the first letter of the first word, including every letter of every word as the eyes move from left to right to the next line and finally to the punctuation mark. "No, dammit, no, it's not right, do it again!" his body screams. Then he quickly glances at the flashing lights on the clock that tick away the seconds, adding another dimension to the compulsive ritual. A dimension unrequested, yet quick to volunteer, that coerces him into letting it be part of his body, to join the "fun." Then he reads the line again. It is still not right. His eyes jump to the clock. He is prohibited from seeing the actual flash but must focus on the clock between flashes. Then he returns to the page for round five of this sparring match with clock and book.

It is touching an object with his right hand and then

forced by an eerie feeling of duress to touch the same object with his left hand, then repeating that ritual time after time until his body tells him, "That's enough, I'm satisfied." He walks away, his energy and self confidence diminished, then suddenly realizes that his body was only teasing him. It really was not satisfied. He returns to the same object and touches it again and again, first with the left hand, then with the right, or maybe twice with the left and twice with the right, or maybe ...

Or perhaps his left hand does not wish to participate and he touches, touches with his right hand, unable to exhale until the need is satisfied. This time his body is not teasing, only temporarily inactive, a rest period that lasts for so little time. He walks away mumbling to himself, "Damn, why do I do it? Why can't I stop?"

This is the father's Tourette syndrome. For others who are plagued with this neurological disorder it may not be as bad, but for many it is worse.

The father does not "officially" have Tourette syndrome. He has never been diagnosed. He has lived for years with these unexplainable, uncontrollable movements and compulsions, the painful muscles and joints and gasps for air when it is impossible to stop.

For years he thought it was caused by stress from his employment. He was devastated and yet somewhat relieved when he discovered through his older son that it was not simply stress but, rather, a complex disorder that is still difficult for him to accept and understand.

The Older Son

It was not until the father's oldest son began exhibiting similar behaviors, the same physical anomalies with which the father had been plagued for a decade, that the family realized something was amiss.

Was the son mimicking his father for some unknown and puzzling reason? Was he also experiencing the same types of stress with which the father thought he had been shackled?

These questions began to be answered when, at ten years of age, the aberrant behavior of the oldest son went beyond those of the father, when the son progressed, or maybe the better word is digressed, from the mere multiple touching of objects, the repeatedly looking under harmless pieces of furniture, to what appeared to the family as a whole new world of aberrations and annoyances.

The oldest son soon began to exhibit vocal tics beginning with periodic high pitched screeches eminating from deep within his body, and increasing in frequency over a short period of time. He then moved on to various motor tics. He became hyperactive, putting an additional strain on the family. He experienced panic attacks that ravaged his energy. His concentration diminished; his self confidence faltered.

At first the family speculated that these motor abnormalities and ritual behaviors were stress related. The vocalizations, however, belied a ready explanation. Even speculation seemed inappropriate.

The older son had already been diagnosed as asthmatic, and the family developed a hunch that perhaps the shrill noise he was making might be associated with that condition since it seemed to emanate from his lungs. It wasn't. But it was at this juncture that the family was pointed in the right direction, albeit, the road to correct and consistent treatment was still long and tough.

It was one of the older son's doctors treating him for asthma who suggested he had Tourette syndrome and that perhaps we should consider taking him to a neurologist.

Tourette syndrome? What was that? It was a condition the family had never heard of. It was an onerous burden in which the family would soon become totally immersed

Finding a physician to treat common viruses, broken bones or even the more complex diseases that plague human kind is rather simple these days. All one need do is check the listings of specializations in the telephone directory. But there is no doctor's name in the phone book that has beside it the words "specializes in Tourette syndrome."

The family thought it was fortunate to live in a moderately sized city that contained three hospitals, one of which was a university medical school hospital. Surely, the family thought, there would be a neurologist somewhere in this vast system of medical providers who would be able to treat the oldest son. The family was wrong.

While the family searched for a physician who could address the needs of the older son, his condition became more severe. The symptoms he had worsened and new ones developed. Since he had been officially diagnosed as having Tourette syndrome, the family began to identify other behaviors that, before the diagnosis, were immune to categorization or association with any specific problem or disorder with which the family was familiar.

The older son developed impaired attention. There were times, though, when he could be found totally engrossed in one particular activity he thoroughly enjoyed. Those situations of rapt attention also temporarily halted any motor and vocal tics he was exhibiting at the time.

Unfortunately, these episodes did not last long for, as soon as he became idle, the motor and vocal tics, the compulsive behaviors and his level of frustration, and that of the whole family, surged with even greater intensity.

Even though the family was confused as to the source and the complexity of Tourette syndrome, and also was unsure of what to expect as each new day arrived, the father was certain of one thing now: there were two members of this family who had Tourette syndrome, and he was one of them.

The Daughter

The family is one that has always taken great pains to investigate and learn about problems, illnesses and occurrences it has encountered as a whole unit or perhaps was experienced by one member.

Upon learning of their older son having Tourette syndrome, the family began the task of reading about this disorder, learning everything they could about it, to hopefully find some sense of order from which they could develop an understanding of what it entailed, and how they could cope with the problems that Tourette syndrome brings.

The family wanted to know what to expect. However, what they were unable to plan for was a second child developing the condition.

The daughter, oldest of the family's three children, had symptoms of Tourette syndrome since kindergarten. Initially, they were barely noticeable. Once the older son had been diagnosed the daughter essentially diagnosed herself based on what she knew about Tourette syndrome at the time. When the magnitude of her symptoms began to increase and the number of symptoms multiplied, she asked for help.

The daughter described many of her symptoms as being pressured from some unknown force to contort nearly every muscle in her body to relieve an annoying itch that permeated each and every deep inner part of those muscles. It might be her leg, her thigh. She would pound the stricken area with her fist trying to beat the sensation out of her system. The next time it might be her back, or her arm or her neck which soon became misshapen by the constant twisting, flexing and turning of her head and neck to relieve the distress that had overrun her. She required physical therapy to correct the shape of her neck.

Then came the compulsions, the ritual, the frustration of finding something out of place, of having to drink a glass of milk — not water or juice, but milk—before being able to go to bed each night.

Phobias developed. Her mind began to race, thoughts circulating through her brain so rapidly she was unable to concentrate on anything before her.

After she was diagnosed, medications that were prescribed to control the tics or the compulsive behavior or the racing thoughts or a combination of all these symptoms created more problems and solved few. Each new medication brought dizziness or blurred vision. The medications made her drowsy or clouded her mind. They blurred her vision and even, in some cases, increased the intensity and severity of her motor tics and compulsions.

The cycle continued, jumping from useless medication to useless medication, resorting to physical therapy to put her muscles, ravaged by severe ticing, back to the way they used to be. It was frustrating for the family and depressing for the daughter.

But the difficulties and uncertainties with which the family was trying to cope were suddenly amplified many times by the discovery that the third child in the family, the younger son, also had Tourette syndrome.

The Younger Son

He was diagnosed soon after the daughter. His symptoms were subtle at first, movements and oddities that were hardly noticeable, in fact things that may not be uncommon in almost any child.

For the younger son, however, they were anything but subtle. In the beginning he was plagued with quick temper and changing moods. He consistently overreacted to sudden changes in routine.

Over a period of a few months he progressed into other symptoms while at the same time the behavior problems abated. He developed alternate symptoms, complex touching movements that interfered with his ability to concentrate and accomplish such things as homework or the simple act of reading a book without becoming extremely frustrated.

These complex touching activities involved the urge to scratch pieces of paper with all the fingers of one hand until his fingertips became sore. He could not stop. He could not keep his fingers from attacking the paper.

It was not particular pieces of paper that coerced his hands to scratch. Any piece of paper that came before him was a target for this uncontrollable urge. When the family went out to restaurants, paper placemats had to be removed from the table so the younger son would not scratch them through the whole meal. He avoided home work and reading because the need to scratch the worksheets or the pages of the book was much greater, the force pushing his hands to paper much more powerful, than the urge to read or accomplish any other act.

When he wrote anything, the letters he put to paper had to be perfect. If they were not, he would have to erase them and try again. Erase them and try again. And again, until he erased a hole in the paper. It took him two hours to do work it took other children twenty minutes to accomplish.

But this symptom passed. Like any person with Tourette syndrome, the symptoms come and go, ebb and wane. Sometimes one may arrive, stay briefly and then be gone forever, only to be replaced by something else just as frustrating, just as unbearable.

There really is no typical case of Tourette syndrome. The family discovered this as each member except one acknowledged being a victim of this disorder. For the younger son, though, gaining membership in this dubious club, knowing he was in the company of his siblings, that he could depend on them for empathy, sympathy, friendship, understanding, did not provide the relief that usually results from such familiarity.

On the contrary, he witnessed first hand the problems his sister and brother had with their tics and compulsions, with their medication, and from this frightening testimony of the anxiety and fear that befall a person with Tourette syndrome, he became fearful that if he submitted to treatment, that simple act would exacerbate the problem.

He refused medication and even denied himself the services of a medical provider who, if nothing else, could possibly give him some support so that he might not have to struggle so hard alone.

The younger son was angry, mad at some unknown force that had burdened him with this unbearable condition. His anger was also felt by every other member of the family, especially by the mother who felt helplessness and frustration in being unable to guide her son to help.

The Mother
The mother of this family does not have Tourette

syndrome. Or does she? She feels she should. Everyone else in her family does. Maybe then she would feel a oneness with the people she nurses when they come to her with their odd movements and sounds.

If the father and only one child had Tourette syndrome, it might be easily argued that this genetic disorder was passed on by her husband somewhere from his family. With all three children having the disorder, it was just too much to blame on one side of the family. Surely, she thinks, her family should bear some of the burden.

She searches her past, her childhood. There were some obsessions and compulsions. There are still some in adulthood. They are subtle, sometimes vague, evidence of some of the same things with which the rest of her family must deal.

What of her mother and father, her brothers and sisters? The mother of this family has thoroughly and carefully examined the lives of many of her relatives, even of those who lived before she was born. Her investigation has yielded some evidence as to the existence of Tourette syndrome in her family. Some of what she has uncovered is purely speculative; there are other instances of tics and obsessions, at one time faint to her memory, but now beginning to show evidence that this condition her children have acquired did not start with her. Rather, she believes that, because all three children have Tourette syndrome, it has been passed to her family from both her and her husband's side.

For the mother there is tremendous strain in trying to cope with the unknown. There is the constant effort comforting, explaining, medicating, waiting for new symptoms, always waiting, and searching for new ways to alleviate them, always searching.

111

Part of her time is spent being a mother to the needs and desires, the trials and complexities that all children experience growing up. But they are multiplied many times over by Tourette syndrome. She spends part of her time as a wife watching her husband struggling with movements and strange behaviors that fill his body with a disease no one has ever officially said he has. The remainder of her time is spent as an individual wondering how it all happened and what will happen next.

The Family

If being typical is the criteria, this family will never be a Neilsen family. There are too many unknowns, very little that is common to other families that are not afflicted with Tourette syndrome. On the contrary, this family is distinctively different, a distinction that is not only a result of four family members having Tourette syndrome, but also the consequence of a need to overcome the disheartening and frustrating dilemma that has penetrated this family's spirit.

To see how the family has overcome its predicament, it is necessary first to understand how that predicament evolved. The circumstances surrounding the development of Tourette syndrome and its attendant factors and events has been a gradual process in which changes in symptoms, feelings and moods have been significantly altered at varying speeds and with differing results.

The physical aberrant behaviors that have demanded responses from this family have already been presented. How the family has been forced to cope, to evaluate and reevaluate, to argue and demand, to console and care, is an even more complex dimension of Tourette syndrome.

Parents of Touretters become authorities on Tourette syndrome out of necessity. When the older son was first diagnosed, as when any child is diagnosed with a condition that is not a part of the ordinary course of childhood, the parents took the son to a specialist, a neurologist. That is what was suggested by another doctor, and the family believed that Tourette syndrome, as it had been explained to them, was better addressed by that specialist.

Little did the parents realize, however, that few doctors, even of those who deal with the brain, knew anything substantial about Tourette syndrome. In fact, the parents quickly realized that the first neurologist they visited knew less about it than the patient he was treating. The treatment was inconsistent. The doctor seemed as if he was in the dark about Tourette syndrome, as if he had to thumb through his medical books each time he was asked a question about it.

The doctor's ignorance compounded his inability to contend with the complexities of Tourette syndrome and act to overcome them. He labeled the older son as being demented. He poured medications down him without comprehending what their results might be. He was unable to conceive of reasons why they were not working. When the older son was having severe panic attacks as a result of his fearfulness of what had besieged him and because of his reactions to the medication he was taking, the doctor did not suggest changing medications, or to take some other logical action that would reduce the older son's anxieties. Instead, the doctor told the parents that the only way to eliminate these episodes was to threaten the boy with a Valium enema if he had another panic attack. The doctor did not return phone calls and did not answer critical questions asked by the parents. Maybe he did not know the answers, or maybe he was inclined to believe that Tourette syndrome was not an identifiable and true neurological disorder.

Some families, unfortunately, never question their

doctor's wisdom. This family did. They contacted a Tourette syndrome support group located in a large metropolitan area located about 125 miles from the family's home. That support group gave the family a list of doctors who were knowledgeable about Tourette syndrome and had worked with Tourette syndrome patients. The family consulted its pediatrician about these doctors and decided upon one who had his office in that metropolitan area. At this point the family's pediatrician became an important source of support and assisted the family in finding the proper medical care.

The 250 mile round trip for each visit was worth the time because the family felt it had found a medical provider sympathetic to the needs of the children and quite knowledgeable not only about the condition itself, but also about new advances in Tourette syndrome research. Despite all of this, however, the family, two years later, changed doctors again after finding a physician closer to home who had done considerable research into Tourette syndrome.

Treatment is not simply finding a medical provider who satisfies the family's requirements. More importantly in fact, it is developing a treatment program that stays in tune with the patients needs, difficulties and uncertainties.

For the two children who have received treatment, the numerous medications that have been prescribed caused many problems including lethargy, overeating, dizziness, blurred vision and diminished concentration. These reactions are caused in part by the inability of the children's bodies to synthesize some medications. However, an additional problem associated with finding the right medication to treat Tourette syndrome is that the symptoms can change or increase in severity sometimes overnight. Additionally, one medication may only treat one set of symptoms while another medication is needed for other symptoms.

For the children of this family, it is a matter of striking the right balance. More importantly, it is trying to determine if there is ever a point in time in the evolution of Tourette syndrome when a balance can be struck. If that point is ever found, and it may rarely be, it most likely will last for only a brief passing moment.

Treatment by a physician is only part of the program. The family found that there was another part of Tourette syndrome that had to be remedied: the perception and lack of understanding from friends and relatives.

The daughter had little problem with friends. She felt comfortable telling her friends she had Tourette syndrome. At first, there were some who were skeptical, but even these friends eventually came around, grasped the nature of the problem and gave an "okay" and went on with their friendships. The two sons, on the other hand, are very uncomfortable, even feel threatened if people find out they have Tourette syndrome.

There was a sense of stability, of assuredness, that resulted from the understanding and assistance extended to the children by the personnel at the schools they attended. Since the three children attend three different schools – elementary, junior high and senior high — the parents had to not only deal with three different schedules but also had to educate at least two dozen teachers, principals and counselors.

The parents felt lucky. Despite some minor problems with a few teachers, most of the people involved in their children's education were eager to learn of Tourette syndrome not only to understand how to provide services to these three particular children, but also to be prepared for others with whom they may come into contact in the future.

Through a Tourette syndrome support group the family helped form, they discovered that not all families trying to find educational opportunity for their children were as fortunate. Principals and superintendents, especially in smaller school districts, were indifferent, uncaring and even rude and threatening. The children in these schools were ignored and one was even expelled.

For the three children of this family, however, the stress of taking their Tourette syndrome to school was minimized greatly.

The family realized they must focus on how the children's condition should be handled in the school setting. That is where the children spend a large part of their day, and it is where they could experience the most social and emotional attacks as a result of their condition. The parents concluded that an informed and compassionate teacher would make a tremendous difference as to how the children cope with Tourette syndrome in the classroom setting.

The teachers, as well as counselors and administrators, play a vital role in understanding what the Tourette syndrome child must contend with as well as in informing other children as to what to expect and how to react, and steering the other children away from negative, condescending attitudes towards Tourette syndrome children. In addition, making teachers informed about Tourette syndrome helps them to more accurately identify other cases of Tourette syndrome and guide those persons toward the proper medical help they need.

The parents made a concerted effort to educate all of those persons involved with their children's education. Initially, this posed some problems because the children did not visually present their tics at school. The parents had problems establishing the fact that the children did have these problems. Though the tics were unseen, the concentration problems were still present. Some teachers were reluctant to believe at first that the children had any problem. But after a great deal of persistence and by speaking to each teacher, counselor and principal individually, providing literature on Tourette syndrome and having follow up meetings to make sure no problems had arisen and to inform them of any changes in the symptoms or medications of the children, the role played by the children's educators proved to be the most helpful to the children.

One important thing the parents realized is that teachers, or anyone for that matter, cannot be expected to react rationally or compassionately toward a child who has a condition that the teacher is not aware of and does not understand. For many who are uneducated about Tourette syndrome, symptoms of the condition are viewed as behavioral problems that elicit a reaction of discipline and sometimes ridicule. The people who educate Tourette syndrome children need to be made aware. That awareness will not only benefit the child with Tourette syndrome, but it will also be transferred to the other children in the classroom. Without education there can be no compassion.

Aunts, uncles and cousins were skeptical and, to some extent, even disbelieving when told that the three children had Tourette syndrome.

Much of this attitude was the result of lack of information. Some was denial. They could not accept the fact that this disorder, known to be genetic and passed from one generation to the next, could have come from a genetic defect. This is a denial that can affect a Tourette syndrome child's self-worth and ability to cope more than any other difficulty or obstruction they may encounter.

The fact that the three children are able to mask many of their symptoms when in the company of other people adds to the doubt relatives have about the extent to which these children are actually suffering. The inability of the family to make relatives understand is a burden they should not have to carry; it is a difficulty that the family continues to try to overcome.

For many physical conditions, disorders or handicaps, society has applied abusive epithets, labels that discriminate against the victim. The antidote to such condescension is to educate the public as well as to foster the self-worth and self-esteem of the person who has the condition or handicap.

There is some research that shows the possibility that Tourette syndrome may enhance certain talents and abilities of those who have the disorder. The family took advantage of this possibility.

The three children had already exhibited signs of certain talents that went far beyond a level of mediocrity. The daughter began dance lessons at age six, eight years before she was identified as having Tourette syndrome. She has since demonstrated an exceptional talent in dance, winning numerous dance competitions throughout the country. She has attended summer training with the Bolshoi Ballet and has been accepted to attend summer training at other renowned ballet schools.

At age nine she began taking piano lessons and within two years was playing at the same level of people who had trained on that instrument for three times that many years. She is an honor student despite the fact that she has missed countless days of school because of concentration problems or as a result of reactions to medication. Both sons have exceptional talent in art, vast knowledge of scientific subjects and are also excellent students, again despite a multitude of problems from their Tourette syndrome that has caused them to miss numerous school days.

The parents have become aware of how interests and activities relating to areas of ability are instrumental in reducing the anxiety and depression associated with Tourette syndrome, as well as almost eliminating the symptoms, albeit temporarily, when the children are deeply involved in an activity to which their talent has led them.

Another way the family has reduced stress is by developing a curious sense of humor about the tics and compulsions, laughing at some of the contortions a body is put through and offering good-humored commentary on the "tic of the week." For the family this is a positive feature of Tourette syndrome. It is a way to reduce the stress and move the children on a straight course to adulthood despite what Tourette syndrome has done to their body and can do to their mind if allowed to fester.

What began as a catastrophe has turned into a family project. Granted, the first year or so of the family's new status seemed like a nightmare. But there quickly developed a feeling of camaraderie within the family. There is never a "Can't you stop that!" because eighty percent of the members of this family can't.

The family continues to experience an evolution. The shadow of Tourette syndrome changes their view of the world and constantly alters and strengthens the intimacy of the family.

Despite all of the difficulties and uncertainties, though they will always be present, the family has had remarkable success in educating those persons that most affect the development of the children. This was accomplished by searching diligently for the right medical care, by consistently and continually promoting the self-worth and emotional strength of the children. By working to diminish the torment and embarrassment and prevent the destruction of self-esteem and motivation, the family has fostered the right blend of understanding, compassion, medical care and humor.

There should be no shame in having Tourette syndrome. What there should be is the opportunity for Touretters to shine, to reach their maximum potential, to be allowed to have lofty goals and to achieve those goals despite any lack of understanding and despite the intrusion of the tics and compulsions and other burdens and afflictions with which they are plagued.

CYCLES OF MISERY

by

Marilyn Johnson

The full blown tragedy of undiagnosed Tourette syndrome is presented here by Marilyn who chooses not to use her real name. Writing about three generations of Tourette syndrome and addictive behavior was not an easy task for her. Shortly after she agreed to write a chapter she called me and said in shock, "The hard part isn't the writing; it's knowing what to leave out." Marilyn left in the most important pieces of her family's puzzle, and watching her grow as she deals with this situation is an inspiration to anyone in a similar crisis.

Adam Ward Seligman

Marilyn Johnson

My motor tics started in first grade. I don't remember any special event or trauma that might have triggered them. I started to rub my chin against the top of my right shoulder. My two older sisters also had tics, mostly of the face, neck and shoulders, but no one remembers when they started – not even my mother. My oldest sister says she can't ever remember being without them. My younger brother had minor facial tics and a problem with stealing. He went from pencils in kindergarten to cars and money in high school. He also became drug addicted in high school and spent two terms in prison later for drug related offenses. Only my oldest sister and I had minor vocal tics — mostly throat clearing.

Over the last thirty-six years I have had too many different tics to list here. The most noticeable and embarrassing ones involved the face (mouth stretching, eye rolling, widening, blinking,) neck (tossing the head to one side) and wrists and hands (twisting, flexing and extending.)

The hardest part was trying to keep still in public, especially at church and school. I didn't want to be "weird." I couldn't explain to anyone why I did these things because I didn't know. I could suppress them pretty well as long as I was thinking about it, or cover them up by yawning, stretching or keeping my hands out of sight, but I knew I was different and that something was very wrong.

The most obvious explanation was that our father was an alcoholic, and we were just "nervous." He lived with us until I was sixteen, when my mother finally divorced him. My most vivid memories of my father were of him coming home late at night when the bars closed. He would talk to himself about how much he hated himself, how he wished he didn't have to think, or how he would kill himself if he had the courage. He would usually end up raging or crying with his head down on the kitchen table or going through the house looking for my mother who would be hiding in a cubbyhole hole inside my closet. When he came home from work without getting drunk he would lie on the living room sofa with his face to the back and read paperback novels until he fell asleep. He never hurt any of us physically. I didn't know until I was an adult that he had tics as a child.

My grandmother told my mother that he made faces. He would sometimes get in trouble with neighbors who thought he was doing it deliberately. He also had a cousin with "odd" movements, but unfortunately, now that I know what questions to ask, no one is alive who can give me the answers.

I found out that Dad started drinking at age nine and that at some point he "grew out of" the tics. My mother says his drinking became much worse after his second tour of duty in World War II.

He was a truly miserable person. I used to listen to him talking to himself and tried to understand. His disjointed ramblings didn't seem to make much sense, but on a gut level, part of me understood the directionless rage, the self-hatred and despair. I despised him, but I knew that something about me was very much like my father. I still can't quite explain it. He knew it too. Once he told me that I was going to be just like him. Now I think that if Tourette syndrome had been recognized sixty years earlier, and treatment had been available, perhaps he would have turned out more like me.

I was desperate for answers. After my first psychology class in high school I was sure that everything would make sense if I just understood enough. I took every psychology and sociology class available to me. I went through every

123

text I could find for references to "tics" or "habit spasms." This was in the mid 1960's and then they were thought to be purely psychological, a symptom of hysteria. One text recommended that children with tics be removed from the home. It also said that eliminating the tics could cause worse problems.

At this point I think I just accepted that I was mentally defective – that my whole family was totally and hopelessly "screwed up." I was functioning pretty well on the outside. Acting normal was a way of life. One benefit of acting is that it helped to control the tics. I've learned since then that there are models and surgeons with motor tics and disc jockeys with coprolalia who have no symptoms while performing.

All my symptoms are at their worst when I am "being myself." I became very intellectual, very objective inside. It was sometime in high school when I realized something else was going wrong. I was too objective. I felt I had no personality of my own. I just reacted to other people. I remember a dream I had where an airliner crashed in the middle of an outdoor stadium as I watched. I felt a terrible grief for all the people on the plane. I woke up relieved that I was capable of genuine unrehearsed feeling.

As friends, I usually attracted self-centered, strong willed people who liked reflections of themselves. But my intellect was always strong and independent. I loved debate. I loved learning. I still don't mind being shown that I am dead wrong because I know that I am closer to the truth. However, intellectual friends are not real friends.

I was very active in and out of school. I ran the school public address system, the bookstore, held office in several clubs, directed the senior play, sang in the church choir, and was active in scouting. I had no "real" friends because I did

124

not feel like a "real" person.

After high school I spent two years at a small midwestern college, mostly because I had never made any other plans for my life and loans and grants were available. The third year I came home and commuted to a local university.

I dropped out of college at the age of twenty-one to marry a very needy, alcohol-dependant man who was even more disturbed than I was. I became a text-book "co-dependant" long before the term was fashionable. Within six years I had three beautiful boys. The first two were just twelve months apart.

I think I began to really "feel" again when my children were born. My maternal feelings and love for them were so strong that it overpowered objectivity. They were bright, active, imaginative and loving. My marriage was not so bright, but I still felt I had been given more than I ever deserved.

The tics started around the first grade for the first two boys. At first it was just some facial tics. I was devastated. I felt I had somehow contaminated what I loved most in the world with "myself"– my "mental sickness." There were also problems in the classroom. They didn't finish their work, didn't follow directions, couldn't handle criticism, cried easily. Both were recommended for classes for the emotionally impaired, though both tested well above average in intelligence and achievement. They didn't seem to have these problems at home. I thought they were wonderful. Our family was so socially isolated that I had little basis for comparision, and because my life was centered around my children I adjusted to their needs and limitations. They weren't prepared for the real world.

Where the tics were concerned, I followed the same advice my mother had been given by her pediatrician –

ignore them. We never talked about them.

I was determined that my children were not going to suffer from my mistakes, so I enrolled in a Parent Effectiveness Training course at the boys' school. The instructor also had a private practice in which he taught Transactional Analysis. My husband was against his boys going to see a counselor but I convinced him it was the only way to keep them out of Emotionally Impaired classes. He did not get involved. He never really took an active part in raising the children. He just brought home the paycheck and criticized what he didn't like. (Consequently, anything that went wrong would be my fault.)

We worked with this counselor for about a year. There was no change in the tics, but the things I learned through him made a major impact on my life and helped me deal with the major crises to come. Basically, I learned that I was responsible for my own life. Simple idea, but very powerful for someone who felt trapped in repeating cycles of misery. The change in attitude didn't happen overnight. It took many years for me to integrate that idea into my life, but the seed was planted.

Unfortunately, our insurance company decided it would no longer cover counselors without the "right" degrees so we had to stop. My husband had handled the idea of our going by ignoring it. The possibility of getting him to pay out-of-pocket was hopeless. I didn't even try.

About this time we changed our insurance coverage to a new HMO that already included the children's pediatrician. The boys were assigned to the only available children's psychologist. What a change! The boys didn't like going to Dr. R. I was required to take them out of school for half a day every week to fit into his schedule. He made it clear that he was not "my" doctor. I felt like the enemy. Instead of being respected as valuable human beings who had problems to overcome, we became "sick" people.

This was a very low period in my life. I had gained enough respect for myself to resent the way I was allowing myself to be treated, but I didn't have the courage or the resources to make the necessary changes. It was clear that my husband was not going to change. By this time we had another son. This one was the apple of his father's eye and he made little effort to hide his favoritism. I was afraid that my husband would commit suicide if I left him. I also had no salable skills with which I could make a decent living.

Its harder to understand why I stayed with Dr. R. for three years. I was still certain that psychology held all the answers. Dr. R. insisted he was making "progress." His attitude toward me merely reinforced my belief that the children's problems were all my fault. However, the tics got progressively worse and more numerous.

My oldest son's tics began to improve, but he was becoming rigid, over controlled and rebellious. He resisted any kind of authority. My middle son was easy-going, sensitive and sociable, but his tics had become so severe that as fourth grade approached, I considered keeping him out of school. Both boys had become targets for the school bullies. At one point Dr. R. recommended that I put them into residential treatment. This was out of the question - even if I could have convinced their father. To me the boys were not a problem.

Their school performance seemed to depend a great deal on their teachers. They both had Mrs. W. for second grade. She was a remarkable teacher. Every time I visited during school her students seemed relaxed and busy, often with individual projects or in groups. Her classroom was not "quiet" like most but she was very much in charge. She clearly liked my boys but she was concerned that they were still often reversing their letters. She also happened to be a reading specialist so she tested them. She found that both were mildly dyslexic, but had already compensated to the point where no additional help was needed.

The boys continued to "work" with Dr. R. until they were nine and ten years old. He got my permission to use hypnosis on them. They both told me years later that they resisted. Mercifully, the HMO started limiting the number of psychiatric visits per year and we stopped going. The boys remember this episode in their lives with great bitterness.

Looking back now, I feel it was a form of emotional rape. They were not there by choice, and the private parts of our minds should be just as respected as the private parts of our bodies.

Near the end of our three years with Dr. R. I ran across a short article on Tourette syndrome. I sent for more information from the Tourette Syndrome Association. A lot of the descriptions seemed to fit my children. I dared to hope that there might actually be an explanation for all this "weirdness." I brought the pamphlet to our next appointment. Dr. R. pronounced the name "Gilles de la Tourette" with a flawless French accent to show how much he knew about it. He indulgently told me that my boys did not have Tourette syndrome

The year before my youngest son started kindergarten my husband was laid-off indefinitely just after finishing his apprenticeship at an auto plant. I was also laid-off from my part time job, but with extended unemployment benefits, we were still comfortable. Taking a lesser paying job would have meant losing unemployment and other company benefits. He eventually went into a depression and stopped looking. He also started having severe panic attacks, but he refused to get help.

The atmosphere in our home was terrible. I felt I had to get my youngest son away from this for at least part of the day, so I enrolled him in the local Head Start program. I had discussed the problems at home with his teacher and she told me about a government grant that was available for non-traditional job trainees. I qualified for the electronics program. I started with one summer class and then took whatever classes were available while the boys were in school.

Meanwhile, I started watching for information about Tourette syndrome. Something just didn't add up. My siblings and I had never seen my father's or anyone else's tics. How could we all have patterned after him? My children had seen my tics, but theirs were much more severe and many were very different, including vocal tics. They also seemed to have less control. My middle son had tics I didn't even recognize at the time. He gnashed his teeth and jerked in his stomach muscles until it hurt and made him feel sick. He underwent a painful operation to enlarge his urethra because no other reason could be found for the frequent leaking of urine during the day.

The age of onset was about the same for the boys and me. We followed the same waxing and waning pattern, but not concurrently. All these things made me think that it could be hereditary. But all the information I could find said Tourette syndrome was not hereditary, and very rare. I had started receiving the Tourette Syndrome Association newsletter, and I finally called and asked for a list of doctors familiar with Tourette syndrome.

I made an appointment for my middle son with a pediatric neurologist at a university hospital. He did a thorough exam and took a detailed history. We finally got a diagnosis of Tourette syndrome. We learned that there was no test for Tourette syndrome and no cure, but he gave us a prescription for clonidine, a medication used for high blood pressure that was also helpful in some Tourette syndrome patients. We were cautioned not to expect any results for at least three weeks.

We started seeing results within days. In a week the tics were gone. He seemed so relaxed and happy. It was like a miracle. Unfortunately, the tics started to return in a few months. The dosage was increased and then side effects became a problem. He became listless and tired all the time, but the tics remained. He had somehow built up a resistance to the drug. Finally, we decided that the "cure" was worse than the "disease" and we took him off the clonidine. At this point in his life he was doing pretty well anyway. He was such a good natured kid that he managed to make some good friends in spite of the Tourette syndrome.

I did not have my oldest son or myself diagnosed. Since there was no cure, there seemed no point in having something in our medical records that might someday be considered a handicap.

When my son was first diagnosed, I was eager to tell my sisters. We had never talked about our own tics. We had never really been close at all. I was surprised to find that they were very skeptical. I thought the news would be a relief, but I think we had learned to ignore the problem for so long it was hard to acknowledge it now. It wasn't until my nephews started having problems that we really started to "talk."

In the eight years that followed my son's diagnosis, I learned a lot more about Tourette syndrome. It is hereditary. Many of my family's problems are also very likely related to Tourette syndrome, alcoholism, drug addiction, oppositional behavior, compulsiveness, destructive inappropriate anger, attention deficit, dyslexia, depression.

Some of our problems are surely the result of living with this bizarre disorder, and the harm we have done to each other through our ignorance. I also now understand why the men in my family have been most severally affected.

I finished my two year degree in four years, went through a divorce and was hired by a utility company. My oldest son is doing well. He is twenty-one now, working and living at home. He has come a long way. He started seeing a psychiatrist on his own a year ago, was hospitalized briefly with depression and is currently on a low dose of Norpramine.

My youngest son started having behavior problems as he approached his teens, especially inappropriate uncontrolled anger. He is also on a low dose of Norpramine. He still gets angry, but he doesn't "lose" his temper. He also has some attention deficit that responded beautifully to medication. He is doing well in high school and is an all-round delightful kid. The few minor tics he has had have been transient.

My middle son is no longer living at home. I was not aware that new medications were available that could help him until, at seventeen years, his behavior had deteriorated to the point where hospitalization was necessary. I didn't know he had been using alcohol and drugs for some time. Perhaps it started as a form of self-medication. He tried living with his father, came back home, was hospitalized again and went through short-term drug rehabilitation. Unfortunately, none of these moves were voluntary and he would not stay on medication long enough to give it a

131

chance. I also suspect the drug use may have made him resistant to appropriate medications.

He refused further treatment and became so violent that shortly before his twentieth birthday I had to make him leave for good. I have talked to him briefly, twice. He says he is living with a friend, working and trying to finish the few credits he needs to finish high school. I can't help him anymore. I can only hope he can make it on his own. I would give anything to go back in time with what I know now.

One thing I have learned from all of this is that medication is only part of the answer for us. It can remove some roadblocks, but it cannot undo all the damage. I am still trying to sort out what is Tourette syndrome from what is "me," what I can change from what I have to learn to deal with.

I recently started attending Tourette Syndrome Association meetings. I have seen families who have dealt with this disorder so much differently. They acknowledge it. They talk about it. They deal with it. I wish I had known long ago that it is something to deal with and not something to be ashamed of. Maybe my son would be dealing with it today.

Early diagnosis, even of a seemingly mild case is so important. Parents need encouragement and support – not blame. Tourette syndrome victims need to know they are not alone – they are not "sick" or "weird." Maybe in some ways it is easier when symptoms are so severe that they cannot be ignored. It was not until I began to meet and talk with others with Tourette syndrome that I really began to believe it might not be "all my fault."

MAKING FRIENDS WITH TOURETTE SYNDROME

by

John S. Hilkevich

In this narrative of the Tourette syndrome in me, I will first tell you about the inner and outer life of a person named John. He was the boy/adult in the years B.P.D. (Before Public Disclosure.) Although I came from John B.P.D. and his gifts and learnings still flourish within my body and soul, we are different entities. John is gone now, though his tracks are still readable. They testify to a legacy of triumph and despair, saintly heroics, and sinful, desperate attempts at trying to feel good, or, at least, ok – a legacy of accolades from his loved ones and the public, and of confusion and pain.

I am still quite fond and protective of John B.P.D. for

John S. Hilkevich

he was a good boy and a good man and did a great job in giving birth, by God's grace, to whom I am now. He blundered at times, and wrestling with the inner demons of Tourette syndrome drained his strength. He died, only a couple of years before this writing, when the voice of his heart uttered, "God, Great Spirit Who Moves in All Things, I give up. I'm done! You take it from here." John's ego made a feeble objection. "Now wait just a minute here, so we can check this out." His heart said, "Shut up; you are done." His ego bled fatally, with the redness, drama and speed of a setting sun. Earth and ego are both swallowed up by darkness. Some Tourette syndrome afflicted persons self-mutilate. So be it ... an ego that claims it can do a better job at running my life than the pervasive Spirit is a good place to begin mutilation.

Some of you may raise an eyebrow of curiosity at the boundary I have created between John B.P.D. and John A.P.D. (After Public Disclosure.) The goal of some Western or modern therapies is integration of our many selves. However, the goal of some Eastern or ancient practices of healing medicine, involving powerful rites of passage or vision quests, is rebirth and transformation. People were even given new names!

You may want to accept how boundaries in Tourette syndrome persons are often diffused: such as between thoughts and speech (30 percent of us exhibit involuntary or compulsive swearing); between our speech and that of others (echolalia, repeating what we just heard); between our actions and that of others (echopraxia, mimicking the gestures of others); between the texture or position of an object and our inner physical tension (obsessive compulsiveness). John often asked himself; "Where does Tourette syndrome end and I begin?" I am still learning to distinguish between what was genetically imbedded in my personality and what I learned.

The earliest childhood happening John could recall is that of encountering chickens in his uncle's coop in Belgium, noisily flying almost right into his face. He was three years old. His mother immigrated from Europe to join her husband in the United States. He had worked his way out of Russia as a teenager with most of his family through a combination of clever maneuvering and luck. French was John's first language and the visual memories of chickens and scale models of castles and the conversation around them still echo in his brain.

John also made strange noises that didn't make sense in French or English. The European doctors decided his tonsils were infected. Years later, John could still remember squirming as an ether blowing mask was pushed over his mouth and nose to put him asleep. Everyone hoped the grunting would leave with the tonsils, but John disappointed them. Maybe that marked the first time that he confused people.

John confused himself about age seven when his piano teacher was in the kitchen talking with his mother. From nowhere, an impulse overwhelmed him: tension built up in his mouth and the only way to rid himself of it was to misalign his jaws and bite down hard. He ran to his bed, throwing his body on it in pain, shoving his face into his fluffy pillow, contorting his mouth and biting down hard.

John was extremely religious as a child. Ritual fascinated him since the first grade and by the sixth he had read the Bible from Genesis to Revelation. Even before starting school, John would feel awed by the presence of a guardian angel. For years John made room for that spirit helper at bedtime, always sleeping on the left side of his bed.

About the same time John acquired many vocalizations, such as whistling. Church services were unbearable, where the periods of quiet triggered the whistling compulsion which he did, feeling self-conscious, ashamed and confused. The grunting gave him sore throats. A holy day was approaching when a saint noted for the healing of throat ailments was honored. John looked forward to the ritual when a priest would hold two candlesticks, one on each side of the throat, offering prayers of healing and protection. John's teacher brought his class to the first service of the day and he prayed for its magic to heal his grunting and teeth grinding. Wanting a double dose, he skipped morning recess to join again a second service and the ritual blessing of throats. By lunch time he moped about, wondering why it hadn't worked. During the afternoon recess he again entered the church at his school only to be disappointed. There was no service. Fear and desperation grew. John kneeled at the altar, crying. After a while it occurred to him that it would all right if he took two of the small offering candies and performed his own ritual at home, if he vowed to pay for them with his next day's lunch money. He kept his part of the deal and kept trusting in God.

John's days of twenty-four hour supervision at summer camp gave him practice in manipulating his schedule to manage satisfying these weird sensations in his body. He would volunteer for kitchen duty every Sunday which would let him get away early from church services. They were too long for his Tourette syndrome compulsion to keep his socks wedged between his little and fourth toe. For months, every hour, he just had to take his shoes off and adjust the sock wedges so it felt tight. And he had to do it so he wasn't noticed.

John's violent head shaking was easy to cover at camp:

he explained to his peers that he had water in his ears from swimming. Adults told him to stop his bad habits. When he tried, his body grew so tense he hurt. His legs shook. He couldn't sit still. His muscles pulled and strained. He had never heard the terms, "hyperactive," "minimal brain dysfunction," or "attention deficit." But he knew something was wrong.

Some nights John apologized to his guardian spirit for all the kicking around in bed. Other nights he slept on the floor and let his spirit companion have the bed. The spirit would not be offended by his distancing himself, unlike some humans.

A story John had been told particularly frightened him. It involved a mysterious, hidden bell that hung between the walls of his house. The bell would ring occasionally. If John was making a Tourette face or gesture, when the bell rang, that grimace would freeze forever on his face. It made sense, as that would explain the strangely contorted faces he saw during strolls through Fairmont Park in old or handicapped persons. His fear of being caught was ever present and he learned to be vigilant.

Colorful and animated was John's world, filled with spirit helpers and the presence of God and he prayed long and hard. (His parents sometimes good-naturedly teased him about getting ready for bed early so he would have time to say his nightly 'mass,' a Roman Catholic ritual whose duration is nearly an hour.)

John's world was also filled with threatening and powerful but unseen forces lurking in bells and walls, of demonic spirits, which were his only logical explanation of those menacing forces in his child's mind. He repeatedly read the account in the Gospel of Mark of the demon possessed man who cut himself with stones and uttered many voices and cried for freedom from it all. John also cut himself, not to end his life but to prolong it, to relieve himself of the inner, unbearable tension just under the skin. He remembers pulling violently at his hair, trying to get the creepy-crawly feeling from underneath his scalp. The creepy-crawlers did seem to flow out with the blood released by scratching his skin with various objects.

John's first novocaine injection at the dentist was a disaster. At first he thought it was an interesting feeling, then his brain crashed inward, pulled by the sensation of the need to feel. He could not tolerate numbness. He had to feel! John knew not to draw attention to those weird compulsions, so instead of poking the outside of his mouth he chewed hard at the inside. No relief! He poked at the inside of his cheek with a pair of scissors and felt nothing. He just had to feel something or he would go nuts! He penetrated the skin, lacerating the inside of his mouth. The taste of blood seemed to dissipate the tension not able to be expressed through the numbness.

Years later John experienced that same penchant for feeling in the most intense fashion ever encountered. Severe back and neck spasms, cave explorations, and long car trips into wilderness areas, combined to herniate a lower lumbar spinal disk. After several epidural injections, CAT scans and months of tremendous pain, the need for microsurgery was established. Given the option of total anesthesia and a spinal block, he chose the latter because he really wanted to be alert during the operation. In the recovery room, he found himself still paralyzed from his diaphragm down to his toes, with no feelings. The nurses assured him the anesthetic would wear off in an hour and John counted each minute. Three hours later he was still numb and going crazy with Tourettic tensions. They could not be satisfied while his brain was active and his body was unresponsive to its transmissions. The dopamine neuro-transmitters were escalating and John had no way to neutralize them as his flailing arms provided no relief. He desperately asked nurses to rotate his feet for a few minutes to relieve the compulsion to move and feel, and they complied for about ten seconds, oblivious to his agony. John's post-operative recovery was riddled with fantasies of taking a knife or scissors to his legs and cutting deep into them until he felt something. That helped a little.

I am an Emergency Medical Technician, volunteering with my local rescue squad, and once was tapped out for a "bleeding" call at 4 AM. I was the first on the scene, approaching cautiously. Central Communication radioed me that police back up would be at least twenty minutes away. As I approached my patient, a young man, he said, with surprise, "Mr. Hilkevich?"

I replied, "Steve?" (Not his real name.) I hadn't seen him for four years. Both his arms were lacerated from the elbows down to his hands, precious blood spotting the ground and my surgically gloved hands. "I'm glad it's you," he told me. So was I. A run sheet on this call would typically list "possible suicide attempt" but it certainly wasn't. The lacerations were not focused on opening an artery. Steve had done that before, along with burning himself with cigarettes. On the way to the hospital we talked about how he didn't want to die. He just wants to live and be rid of some tormenting demon inside. He figured it would come out with his blood, and he did feel relieved. A week later he called me to say he did it again.

Dr. David Comings, in his book, *Tourette Syndrome and Human Behavior* wrote: "Various types of self-abusive behaviors are not uncommon in Tourette syndrome. They include head banging, especially as young children, hitting oneself, licking lips sometimes until they are bleeding and infected, washing hands until they are raw, constant picking at sores, grinding and pulling teeth, and biting their hands, lips, cheeks or tongue. These occur in twelve to fifty percent of patients. *I have a rule that any skin lesion in a Tourette syndrome patient is self-induced until proven otherwise."* (Emphasis his.)

I met Steve for dinner, talked about myself and asked about him. He was riddled with OCD (obsessive-compulsive disorder) symptoms, which interfered with his keeping a job and relationships. Now he knows he isn't crazy. Now he has a new perception.

The gift/curse dichotomy of Tourette syndrome increasingly became a focus of John's conscious attention as he matured. He entered adolescence with the pain of labels such as "Hilke-twitch," misunderstandings, and the physical pain of muscular tensions. Paradoxically, John found out he had to hurt to feel good.

The gift side of John's Tourette syndrome began to surface in his high school years. He devoted three hours a day for four school years to gymnastics and another daily three or four to his academic and personal studies. His reputation grew as a popular student activist and leader, founding one of the state's totally student-run peer counseling centers. Graduating in the top ten percent of a class of about one thousand students, John was asked to make a speech at the graduation ceremony to an audience of 5000. He was the only speaker who didn't need to read his speech. After that no one called him "Hilke-twitch" anymore.

In his private life during those high school years, John experimented with psychological and spiritual disciplines. He meditated, self-hypnotized, prayed, and would leave his home alone once or twice a month to wander in the local woods, praying and listening to God all night, sleeping a couple hours after dawn, and slowly ambling back home. Those times were spent in Tourette syndrome convulsions, storms of muscular explosions and sounds, dissipating the stored energy from the week before ... literally wrestling with the devil.

One of his strategies was remaining very internally quiet. Happiness, excitement, bright sunlight, stress, would trigger a Tourette syndrome episode. For an entire month, John would stay very quiet and keep a tight lid, withdrawing from people and family. He didn't Tourette as much in those times, but he wasn't happy either. John settled for peaceful contentment, although to his loved ones he appeared depressed.

John felt the same as others with Tourette syndrome. His accomplishments were not enough to make life really worthwhile while his inner and hidden demon kept popping around his nervous system. He needed answers too. His childhood magic, rituals and prayers did not deliver him, although they, along with love from family and a tight circle of friends, kept him alive. He felt comfortable with the 'hereafter'; death was an entrance into another life and a chance to leave his Tourette syndrome riddled body behind.

During his high school and college years, John hitchhiked across the United States to hike the Grand Canyon and Rocky Mountains; he would fast for several weeks at a time, cleansing body and soul; he studied martial arts, gymnastics, rappelling and climbing, SCUBA diving, skydiving, fire walking, white water canoeing, caving, hypnotherapy, mystical traditions – pushing his body, mind and spirit past edges where he thought his Tourette syndrome wouldn't follow. But it did, sometimes as a shadow behind him, sometimes as the devil in front.

At one point the devil was in front and had John by the nose. He could hardly breathe, and walking was a chore. He could easily sleep twelve to fifteen hours a night. An interesting article he noticed in a magazine caught his attention. He cut out the report of a "rare disorder" called Tourette syndrome and brought it along to a doctor's appointment near Villanova University where he was attending school. The doctor had heard about Tourette syndrome but had never witnessed it and did not see it in John as he was in his usual, conditioned, public control. Only medical and behavioral history, and not tests, could be used to diagnose Tourette syndrome. He said that if John had it, he recommended a few alcoholic drinks, "when it got bad."

All his life John had been anti-drug, anti-alcohol, and anti-medication, a posture that motivated him to establish the high school peer counseling program. Considering the use of alcohol raised some spiritual questions, which were settled by rationalizations. When it again, "got bad," John tested the advice, bought a pint of rum, mixed it with soda, and felt instant relief. Real and profound relief, lasting for days. He felt normal for the first time. He welcomed invitations to parties where alcohol was served, where he could socialize and enjoy interacting with people, without having to keep his tight lid controls and could feel Tourette syndrome free. It seemed the demon was drowning in toxic alcohol, but John later learned that it was just below the surface, with a mask and snorkel on, and surviving.

Tourette syndrome is like an allergic condition waiting for the right trigger. It is also like having poison ivy all over your body, for twenty years, and constantly being told not to scratch. You can resist for a while, but eventually you give in. So Tourette syndrome is both voluntary and involuntary. "Just stop it! It's a habit!" John could, just for a little while. What is a habit anyway? Is there really such a thing? I have a habit of getting up in the morning and of eating every day. But I can break those habits by a decision. However, I can't decide not to be Tourettic today.

When John was twenty five years old, he lost the feeling in his hands, a sensation of being gloved. The Tourettic spasms in his neck muscles were so intense that circulation and nerve impulses were impaired. John felt relief when the sensations returned after a Friday night party and a few beers. As John grew older, his reaction to a specific quantity of alcohol grew less predictable, in direct relation to his Tourette syndrome level. The tensions behind and in his eye muscles (even during sleep) were so great that he often couldn't focus or see. But after a few drinks, he could see, and breathe rhythmically and shake off the shackles on his body and spirit. Like Tourette syndrome, alcohol was both a blessing and a curse. That is true of a host of drugs used to treat Tourette syndrome. Isn't true of sleeping pills and even food? Of money? Of life? Blessing and curses became less and less of dichotomous opposites and grew more indistinguishable, more integrated, more interwoven.

John thought a lot about where Tourette syndrome ended and he began. Thought intrusions, paranoia, anxiety, the need to check and recheck if he had done something, his nightly but very courageous 'habit,' as a little boy, of checking his closet and under his bed and desk for lurking monsters, his mistrust of numbers (do 5 plus 5 really equal 10?...let's count it again and again) ... was all this Tourette syndrome or was it him?

Then a rattlesnake bit John. He shook up the emergency room staff with his severe allergic reaction to the antivenom the doctors had flown in. His blood pressure was negligible and adrenaline kept his heart beating. His father was asked to leave the ER; John's life was precarious. But he relaxed and surrendered to unconsciousness. His blood platelets were destroyed, those cells whose job is to form clots to stop bleeding. John bled from old wounds and even his gums. Internal hemorrhaging was a threat. Not to John, though, because he was content, except for the fire-burning sensation he felt at the bite site on his hand. For a while he was free from his body, visiting the heavens, until he awoke in the intensive care unit. The first thing he did was to write a note to his parents (good thing the snake bit him in the left hand, now the size of a balloon, as he was right handed): "I'm back and will join you soon. Please don't hurt the snake; he was just being himself and did what he knew to do; nothing personal." His beautiful sister was asked to deliver that note, later becoming a metaphor for my own Tourette syndrome: it does to me what it does, nothing personal. But John still needed to take responsibility for the snake bite and the Tourette syndrome.

Later that night, John heard someone sobbing at the entrance of the ICU. Although it was after visiting hours, he heard a nurse say, "It's obviously his parents, let them in." Thank you nurses, for breaking the rules and allowing that presence of love, that love of God that is ever present, to visit John in the bodily form of his parents that night. In and out of a marriage, in and out of several friendships, I have yet to experience God's love as fully and as powerfully, as in my parents and sister.

The toxic medicine of the snake shut down John's Tourette syndrome. For years following the bite he had no inclination to medicate with alcohol and, as director and instructor of a PEER Program counseling model in a large school district, he created two award winning films for local cable network and program use on alcoholism and suicide. As most therapists do, John was also exploring and understanding his own issues while in the role of a helping agent for others. These were the happiest and most productive years of his life, from the standpoint of his ego and personality development. His spiritual growth had to wait for other intrusions and painful encounters, including what Christian mystics term, "the dark night of the soul.'

Meanwhile Tourette syndrome was not really an issue anymore. Except a casual mention to his parents and fiance, except some grimacing and noise making that really didn't hurt much, except some convulsive neck tensions that were relieved by welcome massages from friends, John's battle with Tourette syndrome was still a personal secret and backdoor issue. He still did not understand it. But he understood the dark night of the soul, the bleeding of the ego parading in many clever disguises, and God's grace.

The dark night passed, and John felt confident, healthy and ready to accept the gift of the ultimate sacrament of spiritual and physical union with a woman he carefully selected after dating many others. And she selected him.

To John, based on the teachings of his Avatar, the Christ, marriage and physical union with a chosen and beloved mate was a metaphor for the marriage of Christ and His people. The bowl of the Native American ceremonial sacred pipe (what Europeans called the "peace pipe") represents the Mother, the Earth, the children of the Creator; the pipe stem represents the Father, the Grandfather, the penetrating force of the infusion of Spirit into matter, the mating of Mother and Father, Earth and Heaven, a man and a woman, God and His people. John welcomed the responsibility of a "Pipe keeper" and respects and honors this Native

American gift that powerfully reflects his own Christian symbolisms.

John kept his virginity for the sacrament of marriage, even in the face of occasional teasing of some males and the sexual zealousness of some females. Not an easy commitment to maintain, as John would have readily admitted. But he knew marriage wouldn't be easy either. One does not need to make vows to carry out an easy task. Love, especially its biochemical sexual component, is not enough to maintain a marriage. Biochemistry fluctuates and sex is readily reduced to an alcoholic type ego pacifier and physical satisfier that can be bought just as well with money. Marriage must be essentially spiritual, and John's spiritual needs were greater than his physical.

The biochemistry of Tourette syndrome and behavior taught John a lot about the biochemistry of love and relationships. Tourette syndrome and its associated fears, anxieties and self-consciousness is a magnificent window into all of human behavior. I believe it hovers at that interface between the physical and spiritual, between the biochemical and its transcendence.

Often equated with sexual love is the Greek word, eros, which is also too often thought of as a lusty love of self. The physical beauty, smell, voice, touch of another person will trigger hormonal and neurochemical discharges into our nervous and circulatory systems that make us feel great. The feeling of "love at first sight." We become addicted to it, a chemical addiction as strong as any other chemical infusion that explains how we can "imprint" the devotion of motherhood in newly hatched chickens onto a basketball and why a newborn stops crying upon being held. It also explains how two people "deeply in love" can suddenly cool their affections when one or both of them no longer get chemically high off each other. That is eros.

I watched our son Jason come out from within his mother. He immediately began crying and the nurse wrapped him up and placed him on a scale. I walked over and softly spoke to him, "Welcome Jason, Hi Jason, I love you. God bless you and your life." Jason stopped crying. Did he stop because he "recognized" my voice as his loving father? Or did he stop because my voice triggered sedative chemicals in his nervous system? When I slept on the floor next to his crib and he cried and I picked him up and he stopped, did he recognize my touch as a loving father or did he crave my touch to trigger neurochemical flows that addicted him to his mother and me? Chldren will learn to love only later... that kind of love that keeps going after the biochemical high stops.

Biochemically, my spouse often induced euphoria in my body and emotions. I wanted much to love her, to love her as God would, no matter how my biochemistry fluctuated. And there were many cherished moments of losing myself in her, when the boundaries between her and me were diffused and difficult to distinguish, as I experience with God. Indeed, marriage is a metaphor for the divine relationship. But paradoxically, we were still separate persons and I knew all along I had my own journey to actualize in this life and she had her's. Our wives and children are not given to us to fulfill our lives and serve as our sources of existential meaning, but to share our journeys and celebrate our diverse paths. Jason, our son, is not my raison d'etre. We must set him free someday. He was born through us but not for us. I trust he selected the best possible parents for his life journey. I know I did.

But the logistics of marriage knocked loudly on my sleeping Tourette syndrome and it soared. Marriage is stressful enough without a neurological disorder. The home must be redefined, the boundaries and responsibilities reshaped, relationships readjusted, time remanaged, perceptions of self redefined.

Tourette syndrome persons mirror others as part of their symptomology. We mimic people's gestures, words, sounds, and ways of walking even. Other persons intrude into our nervous systems and cause biochemical changes in us and we serve as mirrors to them in a way. They, in turn, often feel mocked. People are offended, confused, or angered. I believe even their own personal unresolved and conflict issues are mirrored back to them by us, and so we often become the fall guy. The other person's confrontive responses further trigger the Tourette syndrome person's own conflicts and things roll rapidly downhill from there. Divorce, job loss, family estrangement, lack of loving relationships, social life deficits, school drop out rates, suicidal thoughts, all typically score higher on Tourette syndrome person's data graphs against the control groups in the research literature.

Entering courtship and marriage, John still didn't know enough about where his Tourette syndrome stopped and he began. John didn't know enough to know there wasn't a linear boundary between the two. And in marriage, John would be with another person almost twenty-four hours a day, except those few driving alone to and from work. In marriage, he wouldn't even be alone when he slept. Intellectually, he knew he had to commit himself to his new life-style, and needed to do it gradually. The Tourette syndrome demon raised its ugly head and said, "You are going to have to make room for me!" And the devil raised hell with him. While his wife slept alone in their bed he was sometimes out in the woods, far enough away so she wouldn't feel his kicking and wouldn't hear his groaning, his screeching, his muttering over which he had little control. Sometimes while she slept alone he could attend to his compulsive rituals of cleaning where she had already done so, of typing late into the night pieces of his self exploration, of praying and meditating, and of teasing his brain and that of his friends with philosophical discussions, his Tourette syndrome thought and muscular intrusions subsiding as the bottle of wine they sometimes shared grew empty. But John knew his wife slept very lightly, and probably spent many of those nights trying to make sense of him. He did too. So she really wasn't alone.

John and his wife separated, and his son went with her, although he and their son are only physically separated. Their own pursuits of personal needs overrode the actualization of love, that power that would have transcended and overamped their biochemically and emotionally driven behavior and responses to one another. At least that is what happened to me. But I know that the vow of "for better or worse, until death" fizzled in the toxic intoxication of unfulfilled eros. The personal "dark night of the soul" was re-experienced with dark nights and learned patience and practiced hope and forgiveness. And hope and forgiveness for self and others were gifts to myself for his own mental and spiritual health.

Patience, however, for another did not mean, for John, patience for himself. He had taught his students, his adventure school clients and his friends who asked, that the best gift to provide your world and loved ones is a healthy self. That when you start with changes to the self, the universe must change to hold you. Two people do not each own fifty percent of their relationship. Each own 100 percent. John thought of that as two people holding each end of a rope.

John S. Hilkevich

Each does not control half of it, but each controls the whole thing. Each has equal power to tense or slack the whole thing and each has the power to yank hard and rip it from the other's hand. Sometimes commitments are like that, yanked from your hands, leaving you stunned and empty handed. The empty hand has no place to reach except God's ever present one. And God, that personification of unconditional love, unhesitatingly slides His hand into yours. That is His nature. He can't help it ... so to speak.

John went on a week long fast, secluding himself, alone with his prayers and typewriter. He also self-medicated again, this time with no alcohol but with a huge variety of herbs, teas, amino acids, homeopathic preparations, and stopped eating all meats except fish, some fowl and the meat of animals he would hunt down in his surrounding forest.

He confronted the Tourette syndrome devil and, uncharacteristic of Tourette syndrome persons, John didn't blink. Out of him came a fourteen page autobiographical sketch revealing, for the first time, his experience with Tourette syndrome.

Mark, one of John's best friends, was the first to be told the Tourette syndrome details, and he knew John well. They developed the adventure program together and often spent twenty-four hours on the road providing services and programs from Northeastern Canada to Mexico. Mark knew about John's numbness of his extremities, had heard his grunting, and waited patiently for his mood swings to change. Mark accepted John's occasional seclusion on extended camping trips when John would tell him, "I'll be sleeping by myself tonight just over that ridge in case you need me," leaving him with the responsibility of the camp and our clients. Mark would reply "okie-dokie" not realizing what John really needed to do there: pray and let the Tourette syndrome fly to prepare for his next day of often exhausting control. Mark framed our relationship with unconditional acceptance, despite the confusion John induced within it. I once said to him, "Certainly you must have wondered about the grunting and grimacing and mood swings and peculiar antics throughout those years." He characteristically waved his hand back and forth, replying, "It didn't matter and I didn't care. As my friend, I accepted all of you." Mark is a strong, secure individual, so my Tourette syndrome was not much of a mirror to him. My body and spirit rests secure on his belay line, whether I am on cliff side or on an emotional edge. He never fed into my struggles by trying to figure me out and his solution-oriented approach to our interactions became my own model. I am grateful to him.

Just before I wrote and distributed my story, I was teaching at a community college, providing counseling services at an agency, attending school for my Emergency Medical Technician certification, pursuing a master's degree and servicing contracts with my national award-winning adventure program, Environmental Experiences, Inc. My first graduate program instructor mentioned in class a Tourette syndrome client of his. During a class break I went beyond another edge and revealed my own Tourette syndrome to him. Later that client became the first of many referrals to me. I attended my first Tourette syndrome support group meeting and given video tapes on the disorder, rushed home, watched them and tears flowed. The people on the films were so like me! I found a home in the Tourette syndrome community. Kim, Bob, Debbie and her family, embraced my persona. I bounded beyond another edge with abandon. A couple of weeks before meeting them

I could only whisper to another about this neurological condition and soon after I was circulating my story for the world to notice.

And it did. I received calls from all over the tri-state area in which I live. Allen left this message on my answering machine: "You might as well be my brother because I went through the same thing. Tourette syndrome ruined my relationships and life." Our getting together marked his first meeting another Tourette syndrome person. Allen, like me, managed through meditation, martial arts, alcohol and prayer. He also stretched open in surrender to the Higher Power.

Within that same year, I was asked to participate in a Tourette syndrome study where I donated spinal fluids, blood, urine, MRI shots of my brain, and hundreds of answers to questions ranging from my sexual history to my ancestry. Above all, I met Maura, whose story is also in this book. I was her first exposure to a Tourette syndrome person and we talked about our lives for several hours while IV fluids dripped into my artery. I was struck by her life's congruence with mine, by her spiritual sensitivity, maturity, intelligence and sophistication at her young age. She continues to teach me and mirror me.

Within that same year, Tourette syndrome persons and their families gathered at the top of a 110 foot cliff, instructed and belayed by my good friends Bill and Keith, and went beyond the physical edge that was a powerful metaphor for all the edges we all learned to go beyond. Later we again gathered to rappel down deep into a cave, where the depths of our heartfelt connections were made evident. I was delighted to have had my father join me. May he and my mother live long and well, and my life be an honor to theirs.

Making Friends with Tourette Syndrome

My writings reached the hands and eyes of Adam Ward Seligman, the co-editor of this book, out in California. We are such very different people, but differences don't matter much in the face of connectiveness, for which I am grateful although I don't really understand how such connections are born. But neither do I really understand how a chicken can be born from the slop inside an egg. I am content to revel in awe at life's mysteries. Thank you, Adam, for this project, and enabling me to help channel the vital voice of the Tourette syndrome community.

We are a society in love with labels, and they are useful in categorizing data. You are not your label, however, and you are far more than your dysfunction. (By the way, I am not a "Touretter." Although I am a person with that disorder, I trust you have garnered from my writing that I am a person with many dimensions that cannot be framed with any sort of label.)

If you label me, you will never know me. You will only know your own reflection in the mirror that I will become to you. And you probably won't recognize yourself, thinking that you are seeing me. Just like a monkey. (But don't think about them.)

As a little boy I was awed by the mystical pull of the ancient and sacred. While no one looked, I would rub my hands over the rock engravings at the University of Pennsylvania, trembling a little at the connection I was feeling with powerful and mysterious people. I wondered about them a lot, about what they knew and how they saw the world.

The ancient religions of the east and of the primitives provided valuable insights into my own Christianity and I longed to meet real "medicine" people, mystics and saints. The mystical tradition of Christianity is grounded in the

153

Gnostic. Judaism's mysticism is expressed through the Hassids. The Moslems have the Sufis. Buddhism has Zen. Hinduism has Yoga. The Native American Indians were essential mystical. By mysticism I mean the experience of the divine, not our belief system. Millions of people have fought and died over conflicts with religious beliefs. I don't know of anyone dying over conflicting religious experience.

Religion is a generic term for how we put everything together. This writing of mine is therefore religious. So nothing should be deeper than my religion. It is really how we get along, not what we intellectually believe. It should make a difference in our daily living. It should help us out with our kids, and make a difference during childbirth and funerals.

Tourette syndrome is integrated into my spirituality. It has been both a curse and gift. It has both isolated and connected me. From my youth I experienced a heart felt affinity toward the pain of others, drawn toward arenas of suffering. There is meaning and honor, not in spite of suffering, but due to it. Out of my pain came visions of interconnectedness with the earth and sky and a profound feeling in both my body and soul of being animated by the same Spirit whom the universe cannot contain. With the same intensity of a Tourettic tension, I can feel in my body the hop of a rabbit or the surrender of a hawk in flight to the winds. I physically and emotionally feel the life force gushing from the wound of an injured animal or leaking from a plucked tomato, as so I pray my gratitude as I take life, with mixed feelings, to feed my own. How thin and transparent are the boundaries of life and death!

I now manage my Tourette syndrome with medication, good physical and spiritual nutrition, exercise and discipline, and healthy relationships with my family, friends, earth, career work and Spirit. Now my Tourette syndrome is like a friend who's sometimes a pain but worth holding onto because of what we give each other.

MIN EGEN LILLE VERDEN

(My Own Little World)

by

Christian Melbye Jr.

In 1987, at my first Tourette Syndrome Association conference, I met a family from Norway. Chris Melbye and his son Christian Jr. were delightful and Christian, with his runaway energy quickly gravitated to the center of 'the group' of Touretters that formed. I remember late one night dancing in the disco with Christian and thinking to myself how easy it was for him, despite the language barrier, to fit in with the group.

In later years we have kept in touch frequently despite the distance, and Christian came to visit me in Northern California in 1989. We have shared a strong friendship, and when he expressed interest in writing for this book, I was delighted. In his story we get a sense of cultural

157

differences from our American society, so quick to con-
demn those who are different, to the Scandinavian, which
appears more accepting. But for both Chris and me,
coprolalia presents its unique problems. In 1991, I remem-
ber talking with the Australian Tourette Syndrome Asso-
ciation representatives and one of them asking Chris if he
was aware that he had started, quite suddenly, to swear in
English. "Of course I swear in English here. That's the
language I'm thinking in." Then he muttered something in
Australian slang!

Adam Ward Seligman

If you pick one person, and ask if he or she can tell you one, or some, international words, what do you think he or she would say? Big Mac -Coke - IBM?

These words describe impersonal, boring, "no-mean-ing" materials. Oh, they don't see anything, but their television set, their cars or the weekly baseball game.

What they don't know is that there is a whole world out there, a complete world they have never seen and never will, because they are not part of it.

Yes, you're right. The international word I'm talking about not only describes many different ways of being, but describes a complete world.

MY WORLD – MY TOURETTE WORLD.

Tourette syndrome is one of the few words that you can put under the category "international." If you pick one person, and ask if he or she can tell you one international language, what do you think he or she would say? English? – French? - Spanish? Languages which are useless if you're in the "wrong" country.

The language of Tourette syndrome is the only inter-national language in the world! You've got to learn it, to understand what I'm saying. If you don't know it, I'm more than happy to teach you, all right? If you've been reading between the lines, you've probably guessed I'm not an American.

My name is Christian Melbye Jr., and I'm from Norway. A small, but beautiful country with lots off fjords and mountains up in northern Europe. I have Tourette syndrome. Can you believe that? There are people in Norway who have Tourette syndrome. Tourette syndrome is everywhere, all around the globe. We all do the same, stupid things, over and over. I have the same problems that people in the United States have, people staring at me, avoiding me, wondering what the hell is going on and the problems of not being able to do what I want, without taking caution.

Tourette syndrome can give you so much pain. Talking about normal and abnormal people, you got to realize that people who don't belong in my world, are abnormal. Anybody can join me in my world, but they have to follow the rules. They have to take me as I am. If they can't accept me for what I am, THEY'RE OUT!

So in this chapter, people with Tourette syndrome are normal and will always be. Pain is something everybody has had, sometimes. There is always something that is on your mind. Normal or not, life is full of problems. Small, big, important, less important, problems you can handle, sometimes not. There is always something that is drifting around inside your head.

So there is not much difference between normal and abnormal people . . . EXCEPT: Normal people (with Tourette syndrome) have a problem that they have to carry inside them for the rest of their life. A feeling of not being free. Free to do what your body tells you to do. TO TIC! To tic is one thing, that we can handle. The reaction to the tic can be a disaster, if it comes at a "wrong" time. Can you imagine the reaction in a church when everybody sits there and it's absolutely quiet, and suddenly somebody screams an obscenity?

Going to a dance or a disco is something many young people do. Just to meet old friends and make new ones. Usually that means having fun, if nothing comes up. But for me, and many people with Tourette syndrome, something usually comes up.

Can you imagine the reaction when you're in a disco, talking to a beautiful young lady you want to dance with and after a while you make some strange noise, movement or start swearing? Things that you know you're doing and know you can't control. Things that make the young lady use about 0.5 seconds to grab her things and leave. Things I would rather be without.

Or I'm sitting on a bus, and somewhere behind me there is someone laughing. Probably because of a joke or something, but I will pick it up like they were laughing at me. Laughing at my tics. I have to fight not to make more tics. Somehow I know they aren't laughing at me. I just "feel" they are.

It doesn't look like a big problem to you, but this is an everyday reaction. On the bus, boats, plane, movie . . .

Wherever I go, I'm reminded that I do something that makes people uncomfortable. Which makes me uncomfortable.

I get very upset about reactions to a Tourette syndrome tic, but simultaneously I do understand peoples' way of looking at me.

Because, they don't understand. How can they? I mean, they never will, because they are missing a part of life. Oh no. I'm not calling it a "Tourette syndrome-part," because it would be too simple and this is very complicated, very. Trust me. I've spent many years, thinking about this "part." And to make it completely confusing, I venture to say - "if you don't have Tourette syndrome, you wouldn't know what part I'm talking about."

The part — I still prefer to call it a part — is something that everybody with Tourette syndrome has. I never or very seldom see it here in Norway, but in USA I see it in many persons who have Tourette syndrome. Sometime it can take sometime to locate where it is and sometimes I don't see it at all. But even if it doesn't show, they still have it inside, waiting . . .

I just wish I could be more specific, but all I can say is – when I see it, I know it's there. I can smell it. I can feel it. I can hear it. I guess it's the way Tourette syndrome people are, that make me very impressed with them.

Well, I guess some of you just say, "this is just something he makes up, to make his and the other's Tourette syndrome world more important." Okay, fine with me. Remember one thing, I DON'T CARE, because I'm been around thirty five years, having Tourette syndrome since the age of eight and never (well, almost never) taking notice of what people thought about my way of living or doing things.

Now we're getting closer to Christian Jr. and HIS Tourette syndrome.

As you maybe noticed, I have my own way of coping with my Tourette syndrome. In fact, there is another man, who has the same attitude as I do. Some may say – so what? The thing is, the number of years it took me to get there, is the age of this man. I call him a man, because he acts like one. His name is Kevin and he is fourteen and you can read about him in this book.

Now, what does Kevin do, that makes him so great? He has pointed out four very important things. These four things may seem to you as "no big deal," but it is. Even for those without Tourette syndrome these points are hard to follow. You have to look into Kevin's chapter to see what I mean, but I'll just give you a few details, which are so easy and simultaneously so hard — "BE YOURSELF."

That's it, wasn't that hard. Was it? Try for yourself and you will find out!

I got Tourette syndrome at age 8, got my diagnosis at 20, got interested in Tourette syndrome at 26 and now I'm 35. When I got diagnosed as having Tourette syndrome, it did not change my life. Sometimes I felt sorry for my parents, because they were so happy knowing it had a name and there was an explanation for what I did. You know, the same story most people with Tourette syndrome been through.

But not me.

I'm still trying to find out, if it was my friends, the place I grew up or other circumstances that made me feel comfortable. So comfortable, I did not care if it had a name or not.

As I said it started at 8, when I had conversations with people on TV. I kept "answering" the people on TV. I have a hard time writing sometimes. I just drag the pencil across the paper, so my homework would take so much time. I had to write the page over. I had noises too and sniffing tics. But somehow everybody accepted me and at an early age found my way to enjoy life.

If I could pick one thing that really bothers me it is GOING TO SCHOOL. Not being at school, but I have always done a bad job at school. I'm not talking about behavior or NOT going to school. No, I just never did my homework, did not prepare myself for the tests. I did not mind going to school, it's just I couldn't concentrate on the teacher.

I did all kind of things during my school years, except what I was supposed to do.

Sometimes when people talk to me about their child having problems with concentration in school, I really don't agree. There is nothing wrong with the concentration. The problem is, they just concentrate on the wrong thing.

Well, I didn't do well in school, but did my Tourette syndrome bother me? NO!

The only thing that bothers me, is the situation. The fact that it did not make any problem for me, I wonder why and I always will.

As I got older there were more schools, more "funny" situations. "Thoughts about jobs," you may say. No, not one thought. That wasn't included in my Tourette syndrome-world. And I still don't have a real plan for my life. Of course occasionally something like marriage or family crosses my mind, but it is still just me and my Tourette world.

I definitely would like to share my life with somebody and have some to take care of, but I don't take life too seriously. Sometime I feel I'm a "chicken," who's blaming my Tourette syndrome for being single. Even I have one very important rule in life and I think it's important for everybody with Tourette syndrome. Don't let your Tourette syndrome stop you from doing things. (I know Kevin, that was part of your second point.)

Well, marriage or not, my life goes on at the same speed, action, fun, friends, happiness. . . .

One thing that pops into my head. Sometimes it can be real hard to remember things you did yesterday. I need "help" to remember what I did. The situation can be very frustrating at work.

My work is to install stereo, cellular telephones and alarms in cars and boats. If a costumer comes back the next day and needs some extra help or instruction, I sometimes find myself not remembering what I did with his car the day before. Very frustrating, believe me. I know it's a part of me, I can't help. So. . . . I've got to keep on going, I can't stop now.

You got to fight. A fight that EVERYONE with Tourette syndrome has every week, every day, every hour, every minute, every second, every. . . .

A fight that will continue the rest of our life, but we can't just sit still and wait for a miracle.

I know, there are some out there who don't think they are fighting, they just sit there, not doing anything. They have given up. But take my word for it, you're fighting. When you wake up in the morning, you continue the fight from the day before. If you feel that I'm wrong and think your situation is hopeless and don't see any reason to fight back, do me a favor, will you. Talk to me! Write to me! Let me make you realize what is out there. Out there waiting just for you.

I'm not educated in Tourette syndrome. I'm not a doctor. I'm not even an American. I just know how it is... That's all. Do we have a deal?

How can I tell how it is to have Tourette syndrome? Tourette syndrome is something that controls your whole life. You have your Tourette syndrome twenty four hours a day. It never stops. I don't know how it is NOT having Tourette syndrome, so how can I tell how it is to have it.

I can tell how I feel and what's bothering me and all my problems. I can imagine how it is, not having Tourette syndrome. My life has given me a lot. If people tell you, they know how it feels to have Tourette syndrome, without having it, they don't tell you the truth. They cannot under any circumstances know how it feels. We all know that.

One thing, having Tourette syndrome, is that you're more understanding about other peoples problems. You accept more. You want to help all kinds of people, whatever the problem is. Because you see "problems" from another view. From a view, very few people see it. Sometimes I don't think about it, but suddenly I realize there are other people who have problems too. And if I have mine under control, I'll try to help.

My Tourette syndrome life is a life filled with humor. Much humor. Sometimes. . . . maybe too much. I don't know, but it could be a way to survive. Some sort of escape from the world that just accept their own world, not mine.

My life is not boring. And I don't think my friend's find me boring. I remember at the very last day in McLean, at the Tourette Syndrome Association Conference in 1991, I was having dinner with Adam (you know him) and Paul (from Australia) and suddenly Adam asked me, "Are you hyper?"

Never has anybody asked me a more appropriate question. Well, I do know I sometimes talk too much, but "hyper?"

YEAH! AFTER SPENDING THREE MINUTES THINKING, I KNOW I'M HYPER!

Thanks Adam! I OWE YOU ONE!

Imagine, I was thirty-five and two days before realizing I got something else than a "typical" Tourette syndrome. I'm telling you - "life is full of surprises," believe me.

Surprises for me are a keyword and they are what keeps me going. People never know what I'm up to. I don't

165

Christian Melbye Jr.

"make" surprises. They make themselves.

I remember, after the Tourette Syndrome Association convention in 1991, walking in Manhattan about three o'clock in the morning with a friend who gave me a new perspective on the person Christian Jr. And for the very first time in my life, I realize, I will never be able to explain to anybody who I am. I guess it hasn't anything with my Tourette syndrome, but what comes with the Tourette syndrome.

My life has been limited by my Tourette syndrome. But the sun has shined on me too, sometimes. I do know, that because of my parents, my life went on much easier than most people with Tourette syndrome. They have always accepted my way of being. Whatever happened, whenever it happened or how it happened, they always backed me up. When I was younger I didn't think to much about it or what I was doing. I just didn't think about it. Today I understand how lucky I have been, and I'm very grateful.

My closest friends are in the Tourette Syndrome chapter. I do not understand why I was never asked about my tics in my younger days. Even at the time when my odds weren't too good.

Like in 1969 when I moved down to the south part of Sweden (the country next to Norway, with a different language.) I moved with my parents and had to make new friends, go to a new school and learn a new language. Fortunately the language didn't make it to difficult for me (the difference between Norwegian and Swedish isn't that much.) I was amazed at how smoothly things went.

I went to a different school without any big success. I never did my homework and it didn't take long before I didn't care about if I were the one in my class who always

166

had the lowest result on tests. Of cause it did matter, but I learned to live with it and I guess that is the thing I mostly regret in my life.

My problem in school was not that I wasn't accepted, ooh no. Somehow everybody took me for what I was, but my concentration was real bad. And because I accepted this, I did not really try to make it better. I just went to school, sat in class with my Tourette syndrome (which didn't seem to bother anybody) got home and went out with my friends.

I have gone through so many different levels of education, I would be more than happy, if I knew half of what I was supposed to know. So many years of finance education, engineer education, sound-engineer education and lots of other courses, I've been through. So many years just flushed down . . .

From the time I was 17, I've been spending thirteen years trying to learn something from the school system.

But I learned a very important thing. I've been lucky. Lucky to be accepted by people who became my friends. Lucky to been able to think with a clear head, just because I've been accepted. After I met so many different people with Tourette syndrome, around the world, I wish with all my heart that people could understand what difference it makes being accepted or not. I have been listening to many people with Tourette syndrome, talking about their experience in life and I sometime I feel a little bit ashamed. Ashamed to have been so lucky in my childhood when so many had such a hard time. Sounds silly, doesn't it?

It seems like my friends accepted me whatever I did and I guess that is how I made my own "world." A world where I did what I wanted to. Something that helped me with my Tourette syndrome.

When I said I do the same tics as Americans, including

Christian Melbye Jr.

coprolalia (involuntary swearing) I can hear you ask me one thing, "Yes, I do swear in Norwegian." That is the same thing all over the world.

I would say it's fascinating, if it didn't make so much trouble for me.

You know, many tics are impossible to hide, but coprolalia is so difficult for me to hide, and it's so unacceptable.

One of the hardest times to have coprolalia, is when I'm with small children or young kids. Not because they stare at you, but it's difficult to explain so they understand. In a young fellows ears, swearing means just one thing. Something they learn not to say, ever.

When I try to explain it to my youngest niece, I know she doesn't understand it. I can see her accepting my explanation, but I can see it in her eyes, They just say – hmm.

When it was explained to me why I did these movements, back in 1978 when I got my diagnosis, it did not make any difference for me. Of course for my parents, who had dragged me all over the country to find out about what I was "doing," it was a relief. We happened to see a doctor, who had just arrived from a conference for Rare Diseases in the United States. He had picked up something about Tourette syndrome and was then able to give me the diagnoses.

For me, it was a day like every other day. I didn't need any answers, because nobody asked any questions. I was just like everybody else. But I did have a lot of tics. I do hope my parents realize what they did and still do. To accept me the way I am and the things I do is something that far too many parents don't know how to do. To accept their child.

Later, in my "older" days, Tourette syndrome would make a bigger difference in my life.

In 1986, my parents and I started up Norsk Tourette Forening from scratch. Believe it or not, we did not know anybody with Tourette syndrome. We just sent out invitations to a Tourette syndrome meeting and gave it to some doctors who had some Tourette syndrome patients. That very evening we were suddenly eight families with Tourette syndrome and nobody knew each other. That was the beginning of the Norwegian Tourette Syndrome Association. Since then we have about 400 members (1991) and I started to realize that the number of cases of Tourette syndrome is in Norway like everywhere else in the world. Of cause it doesn't make me too happy every time we get a new member, which means there is another one out there with "problems," but it also means we can give these "new" Tourette syndrome-people a better start on a new life and give them a change to meet other people with Tourette syndrome.

Meeting people with Tourette syndrome always give me a good feeling. And when I went to the United States to join the Tourette Syndrome Association National Congress in Cincinnati in 1987, I was not sure what to expect.

Well, my parents and I had a plan. My mother and I would go shopping while my father went to the sessions. We didn't really see the view of the whole conference. We did not pay too much attention to it. More like a vacation. Boy, were we wrong. In one moment, I was in a huge family. A family whom I felt I had known for years. I can't remember if it was their Tourette syndrome or just their friendly way that appealed to me. When I use the word "family," it's just what I mean. We suddenly became a group of people who never met before and we totally freaked out. I'm not sure what the rest of the guests thought, but looking back, we were running the whole place without taking any notice of the rest of the people. Even after my third congress (in 1991), I feel that the one in Cincinnati was the breakthrough and then we were improvising a lot.

Then, young adults weren't a reality for the national Tourette Syndrome Association and they were not really prepared for us and I think that is what made it so very special. I very often think back to the time when I met "the Crazy People in the West" and enjoyed every minute at every congress, when new people "join our group."

What is it, that brings people together, the way it brings "us" together?

The total freaking-out ideas coming from Sharon, to the always smiling and laughing Eli. From the friendly Tim to the multi-knowledge Orrin. The list can be very long, but the list is not important itself. The important thing is, that I hope "we" show people, young or old, that Tourette syndrome does not stop us from doing things. Not for one day. There are of course, some people that grow deeper in my heart. I guess it's not a secret that Adam is one person I was very lucky to meet in Cincinnati, a person with a lot of things going for him. You can't stop him. And he is always more than happy to share it with you. So I'm happy to share my Tourette syndrome world with him. Thanks Adam! Although the Tourette syndrome is similar in United States and here in Europe, there is for me a very big difference. Here in Norway and our association, my thoughts about Tourette syndrome are more like a job. I feel that I'm using all my time helping others with their Tourette syndrome, which of cause is very nice.

But as soon I put my feet on the American ground, meeting the Tourette syndrome people in the west, it's all about our Tourette syndrome. So much more relaxed. Something that is a feeling I cannot so easily explain for you.

As a European, I've traveled a lot in Europe and in the USA. I have met many different people under different circumstances and there is something I have spent much time thinking about. I have found that people with Tourette syndrome are very warm and tender. Always trying to help each other as long as possible and they have a lot of emotion inside. It has of cause something to do with our "problems." We have it everyday, always I can never escape from my "problem." A matter of fact, I very seldom use the word "problem," because I don't like it to see it as one. It's just that sometimes I have to use a different language to get myself understood.

For me Tourette syndrome is much more than just tics. Tourette syndrome is a part of me.

How is it, not having Tourette syndrome? I don't know. I don't know how it is to live without Tourette syndrome.

If somebody could take away my Tourette syndrome, how much of me would be lost? Would I pay the price to get rid of my Tourette syndrome? Or do I prefer to keep on living a life that has given me a lot, even with Tourette syndrome.

A life full of excitement, lot of fun, good times and bad ones. When I look around me and see people, who don't have Tourette syndrome, and look at their situation, their way of living or their behavior, would I change my life with theirs?

There are always times when I think everything is hopeless, everything is against me, when I'm having problems enjoying life, thoughts that everybody has, sometimes.

I would not change my life with anybody. I can't have it all!

RHYTHM MAN

by

David R. Aldridge

If I hadn't met David Aldridge, I probably wouldn't be a writer. When we met in 1979, he talked so much about the healing power of drumming that I had to try it. As I learned to play drum set and learned the control that aided me in learning to suppress my Tourette syndrome, David was often teaching me new concepts. My first sale as a writer was to Modern Drummer magazine, an article about drummers with disabilities. David was among those I interviewed. At that time he was playing with Arthur Brown, who had a series of hit records in the 1960's. At other times in his career David has auditioned for Frank Zappa, and played on several independent artist recordings. David and I became the world's first all Tourette syndrome writing team in 1991, pitching stories to Star Trek – The Next Generation, and writing articles for Drums & Drumming and Modern Drummer. We

173

David R. Aldridge

spent several exciting weeks in Los Angeles in early 1992, meeting with producers, story editors and jazz musicians, as we pursued our twin muses of writing and music. I'm very pleased to have David's chapter in this book. I hope you enjoy it.

Adam Ward Seligman

I've been banging on car dashboards since I was six years old, following and flowing with rhythm until it poured out of my ears. Perhaps it is just coincidence that Tourette syndrome also entered my life at age six; I always thought it was just due to the bicycle crash in front of the neighborhood church. Twenty-six years later, I often wonder if it wasn't more along the lines of Providence.

Rhythm and Tourette syndrome have been intertwined from the first day I found that drumming on a table could mask my jerky hand, leg and neck movements. Playing "Wipeout" on the grade school lunch table was a way to entertain friends and briefly wow and entertain the not-so friendly. However, drumming and rhythm soon became much more than entertainment.

This newly found masking movement actually harnessed my unbounding energy, directing it into an orderly flow. It had also become a socially acceptable form of movement. This "permission to explode" let me tap into vast reservoirs of sounds and physical sensations, and I realized that my destiny lay clearly before me. I was to become a rhythm man.

I started formal drum lessons at age nine from the local music teacher's son in Charlottesville, Virginia. Ken Berry was a teenager trying to make a little gas money by teaching young students the finer points of snare drum playing and reading basics. My attention deficit and learning problems made reading music an exhaustive chore. It soon became obvious to both of us

174

that what I did best was just play the drum and let myself go.

There is a moment from that first lesson that will stay with me forever. We were almost done, and I asked Ken if I could play something I was hearing in my head. He nodded, and I tried to reproduce a simple little march riff. It came out rough, but it was a direct connection, a sign of things to come. I could feel that one day I would learn to harness the enormous energy of Tourette syndrome and control it like a high pressure fire hose. In this case though, my fire hose would pump gasoline, and I'd be burning down music houses.

On my tenth birthday, my mother bought me a snare drum, and I joined a local drum and bugle corp group. We drummers stood side by side, cramped in a small room, banging out rudimental patterns on long planks of wood in place of real drums. I was learning the basics of corp marching drumming, something that I'd use later in high school to help me become one of the top young players in Delaware.

I was very attuned to touch, probably from my body going berserk all the time and me trying to control it. It seemed that in some ways, the more aware I became of my body and the muscles, the more they betrayed me. My symptoms had included neck and head jerking, blinking, facial grimaces and some vocalizations. Fortunately, I had been spared the coprolalia (involuntary yelling of obscenities.) However, stomach and diaphragm contractions, leg and hip spasms and arm/shoulder movements had given me a physiological roller coaster ride I didn't care to continue.

Every impact of the stick became a feedback signal, and my hands learned very quickly how to make the sticks dance. I also began to associate sounds with movement patterns. If I heard a drum pattern, the signals would leap from my mind to my hands. It was as though they already knew what to do. I was beginning to tame the demons in ways I barely understood.

175

David R. Aldridge

The nature of obsessive compulsive behavior baffled me as a child. Sometimes when I would try to drink from a glass, I would first have to touch my upper and lower lip. If I were walking and turned in one direction, I HAD to turn in the other direction an equal number of times before being able to continue. OCD had a definite effect on my drumming as well.

The same driving sensation would make me hear rhythm patterns over and over in my head, a series of obsessive repeating thoughts. The associated movement signals would run rampant through my synaptic network, and they begged to be heard on whatever surfaces were available. The begging only grew louder with time.

My hands and feet would tap incessantly at the dinner table, and my mother would constantly chastise me for banging and disturbing everyone. I could not convince her that something far more than random cacophony was taking place on the plates and in my mind. I was forming the foundation of my ability to explore rhythm.

Pillows, cookie canisters, cardboard boxes . . . anything that would accept the impact of my drum sticks became fair game. I memorized the classic cult sixties drum solo "In-A-Gada-Da-Vida" by Iron Butterfly, and I used to knock the stuffing out of four colored sofa pillows to make the different sounds as I sang along to it. Pencils and different size tumbler glasses were also prime instruments in later years. The urge to play and the desire to release the endless tension of Tourette syndrome fed on each other like fuel on fire.

My twelfth Christmas was the best ever; that's when I found my new shiny blue sparkle drum set hidden in the trunk of our car on Christmas Eve. It was also the last time I ever went looking for presents. Some surprises are best kept undiscovered; the magic must be preserved.

I'd abandoned the idea of further formal lessons because I

just couldn't sit still and concentrate. Too much music and too many sounds were screaming through my head, and I had to allow them room to breathe. I concentrated on learning how to get my hands and feet to play as fast as possible to be able to capture the fleeting ideas. Mastering speed also provided an even greater outlet for the tension. Musicality would develop many years later.

I successfully passed the seventh grade jazz ensemble audition with the understanding help of Bernie Kosk. This band leader realized I needed to play, and I was the kind of kid he liked. No parent was making me take band to get culture; I *wanted* to be there. The school's green sparkle Ludwig drum set was the coolest thing on the planet as far as I was concerned, and I was destined to become its captain.

Keeping time was difficult, and my reading was terrible, but Mr. Kosk didn't to seem to mind too much. He knew I was a fireball, and his challenge was to direct that fire into the other musicians. There was another drummer in the band, Jim Shepeard, who used to sit next to me and read the music for me. Jim would tell me when to stop and start, and I owe him for that. Between the two of them, I managed to play in front of people and feel the thrill that more kids ought to know. My movement disorder was not only being accepted; it was being met with applause.

The teasing that invariably accompanied Tourette syndrome affected my musicality as well. I eventually decided that if people were going to stare, I was going to give them something to look at that they would not forget. My rage and adolescent hormones teamed up and created a formidable demon, a drumming maniac in a thirteen year old's body.

I became obsessed with drumming, spending hours behind the set unleashing torrents of rage and anxiety. These sheets of kinetic sound ripped through the walls of my bedroom out into the unsuspecting neighborhood, often drawing a crowd of curious listeners. They were getting a small taste of the inner hell I was trying to harness and release safely.

My drum set grew to fit my need to explore tonalities, and my hands and feet reached out to new dimensions. I began listening to a wider range of music, incorporating jazz, rock, funk, soul and anything else I could get my hands on. Each style was a variation in basic movement, and that was what music had become to me.

I entered Glasgow High School's music program under the watchful eyes of L. Jerome Rehberg. This incredibly patient band director encouraged me every step of the way, promoting musicality and humanism over competition and ego. Since no one at the time (myself included) knew I had Tourette syndrome, Mr. Rehberg's understanding and openmindedness meant a great deal. I owe him especially for introducing me to jazz.

Jazz captured my ears, with its syncopation (unexpected accents) and improvisation. I loved the pops and cracks, the free flowing motion of time over variations of time. My body swam in the river of rhythm, quite at ease with the unexpected. I'd found a normal environment to call home . . . and there was not a tic from me in the house.

By age sixteen, I'd struggled through classes with little academic ambition. Had Hank Levy not come into my life, I'd probably be in a rock band somewhere playing top 40 hits on a Holiday Inn circuit. Hank was a jazz instructor from Towson State University in Towson, Maryland, outside of Baltimore. He'd won a government grant to introduce jazz to the high schools, and he was bent on teaching us how to play music in odd meters. This was the premier turning point in my life as a drummer and a thinker.

His music didn't go "1-2-3-4" like most Western tunes. Hank was a writer for big bands led by Stan Kenton and Don Ellis. These men, like Hank, were pioneers, reaching out beyond the standard definitions of jazz. Their music was often counted "1-2-3-4-5," or "1-2-3-4-5-6-7, " and the first time I played this stuff, my body lit up like a Christmas tree. It had NEVER moved or felt like this, and the patterns soothed my Tourette syndrome like nothing I'd ever experienced.

About the same time, jazz guitarist John McLaughlin emerged on the music scene with his Mahavishnu Orchestra. He combined odd meter music with the sophistication of jazz and the unbridled power and volume of rock. To me, it was absolute Nirvana. His drummer, Billy Cobham, was a human Gatling gun turned loose on a drum set. I copied his style and let my Tourette energy loose with no holds barred.

I had discovered "fusion," the 1970's jazz answer to psyche-delic rock where just about anything went. My body had permission to do whatever it wanted, as loud and fast as it wanted. This was a roller coaster ride I didn't mind, because I was directing it. The audience didn't seem to mind too much either. They enjoyed watching a long haired, hands and feet flailing teenager go berserk in a controlled sort of way. And I never tired of hearing the applause.

I resumed drum lessons to improve my reading and coordination. The next two summers were spent attending the Stan Kenton jazz clinics at Towson State, becoming exposed to a new world of drumming. Peter Erskine was Kenton's drummer at the time, and I learned a valuable lesson about Tourette syndrome and musicality from him. To date, most of my drum soloing had been an unrestrained purge of burning energy, striking out at drums and cymbals like sparks in a fireworks warehouse. One afternoon with Erskine really turned that perspective around.

There were about twenty drummers in a room, and Peter paired us up to have a drumming dialogue. We were to play back and forth, have a conversation, learn to make a musical statement. Up to that point, I'd just held my breath through songs where I could solo, just waiting for the chance to cut loose and impress people. That day, I felt no different than I had a hundred times before.

I began to play along with a guy, and pretty soon, I was exploding all over the place, lost in my own Tourette escape world. When I was done, the room was silent, not a sound I was accustomed to. Their looks said it all. I'd made a fool of myself, just making a lot of noise and not a whole lot of music. That lesson stuck with me, and from then on I decided to make real music on the drums, not just create a display for self-indulgence. I would learn to listen.

By my senior year, I had refined my playing and my behavior. The nervousness was hard to control, but playing jazz gave me the maturity to approach it with. Friends and teachers had finally become accustomed to the wide range of symptoms that were my show. Learning to play and compose on the piano helped soothe the stress level in places where drumming couldn't, and I felt blessed to have so many musical gifts. My mind was set on going to Towson to study more with Hank Levy, and music seemed like the chosen path.

I'd landed the first chair in Delaware's All State Symphonic Orchestra and Jazz Group, and I'd won the lead drum seat in the American Youth Jazz Band. This was a tri-state honors band that included a couple of today's premier jazz musicians. Things were looking pretty good for a guy who couldn't sit still, but one mountain remained to be climbed. I was determined to leave an artistic impression that would be talked about for a long, long time to come.

The final concert of the year was coming up, my last chance to play with high school friends in front of an audience that had become familiar over the last four years. I had a solo in one of Hank Levy's songs, called "Quiet Friday." It was anything but that, and Hank liked my nervous energy being channeled into his music. My jerky movements stopped when I played, and I think he realized how therapeutic music was for me. I felt that his works were of particular value, and I wanted to set this one on fire.

For weeks, I explored ideas to throw into the drum solo, things I thought were both musical and explosive. The day before the concert, I sat behind the closed auditorium curtain, imagining the audience hidden behind the bright lights. I wanted to play to them, give them a piece of myself and my energy. It would be my last chance to give them something to look at. After all, hadn't that been the goal just a few years before? The teasing, the emotional scars, the pain and loneliness could all disappear for a few moments when I was on my own behind a drum set.

The next night I was more nervous than usual. I held it in, trying to go very deep in mental preparation. The curtain rose and we played through all our songs, saving "Quiet Friday" for last. We played the soft intro, and then things sort of went blank. The tempo started off MUCH faster than we usually played it, too fast for me to play the ideas I'd spent weeks working out. I felt like I was on a runaway train speeding out of control toward a black abyss that called, "Okay David, let's hear what you can do with this." Someone had pushed me off the edge of a slalom ski jump, and I was about to leave the ramp.

The music stopped, and something in me took over that I barely understand even fifteen years later. My hands and feet felt a surge of adrenaline that sent chills all over my body. I danced around the cymbals, listening to their echo in the 1000 plus seat auditorium. Musical ideas were coming out of nowhere, from a place I'd never been before. It was a stream of consciousness and fear, gushing out of my limbs in a perfectly controlled flow of unrestrained energy.

The solo had form and style, all being improvised on the spot, and it was LOUD. Cymbals and drums exploded in combinations I didn't know existed. My body had controlled me for years, but for these brief nova-like moments, I directed the fire out toward the audience with utter conviction. The hall echoed with thunder that stirred souls and sent chills into their spines.

I did to the audience what my body had done to me most of my life. They were seeing - no, 'living' the Tourette experience at its zenith. Drumming transformed me and became a vehicle to show how a disadvantage could become a larger advantage than I'd ever imagined. I brought things down to a hush, blew them up again, throwing in flams and riffs that were completely unexpected. A soft roll here, a KA-BOOM there, all within the musical moment. The demons wanted out, and I let them go with a vengence.

The solo ended with a barely audible cymbal roll being brought to a deafening roar that filled every square inch of that auditorium. The music kicked in, the band took off, and I could hear the shrill whistles and thundering applause through it all. The experience took both audience and player to a place neither had been before, and I've never been more in the moment. That magic night, I harnessed the fear and hurt, the hope and pain of my soul; and if I learned nothing else, I saw that Tourette syndrome had a side to it that I'd spend the rest of my life trying to get back to and understand.

That night, I became a Rhythm Man.

IN THE GROUP
LIFE AT A TOURETTE
SYNDROME CONFEENCE

by

Adam Ward Seligman

"The person I can't get out of my head," Elisabeth said to me at three in the morning, "is Candy. I see her face, etched with pain, and I want to do something for her, but I know I can't."

Candy was one of the twins from Atlanta. She and her sister had very severe Tourette syndrome, and for one reason and another, she represented the worst case scenario of what Tourette syndrome used to be. She was isolated and incapable of leaving her house. She could not stay in school or work without the fear of rejection or of discrimination. She also felt terribly guilty about her symptoms: you could see it in the way she apologized for her tics, even at a Tourette Syndrome Association conference.

The same question was on everybody's mind. If Candy was this bad, what was her sister at home like?

"The other face I keep seeing," Elisabeth told me that night, "is Shane. His symptoms are as severe as Candy but he is such a different person."

"He's a kinetic sculpture, Tourette syndrome as an art form." I suggested.

Elisabeth nodded. "He is the beautiful side of Tourette."

Candy and Shane, two sides of the same coin: severe Tourette syndrome. What were the reasons that one survived and one suffered? With that question lies madness.

When people with Tourette syndrome started getting diagnosed in large numbers, during the 1970's, one issue which wasn't addressed at that time was what would happen to them. We were the first generation of correctly diagnosed Touretters and possibly the last to suffer years of misdiagnosis. We were fortunate and in the right place at the right time. But, as I told Christian, from Norway, we were also a lost generation. Our story was going to be the most unique in the history of this disorder, because after us, nothing would ever be the same. Ten years from now the correctly diagnosed children with Tourette syndrome would be running the show and our generation would possibly be an embarrassment to them with our emotional issues.

There were over 525 people registered at the 1991 Tourette Syndrome Association Leadership Conference. My guess was about 100 had Tourette syndrome in some form. There had never been a larger gathering of people involved with the disorder and for three days we lived and breathed the disorder with both tragic and comedic results. Images flicker through my mind, faces and comments, all mixed up with an after conference collection of tics and urges.

Elisabeth doesn't have Tourette syndrome. She has a brother with it and she works with children with Tourette syndrome in the Detroit chapter. Through our conversations and emerging friendship I got to understand the point of view of the normals at our conference. As we sat talking late Saturday night I kept on touching her knee or her shoulder. The topic of what had become an epidemic of touching tics came up.

"Somebody was complaining that it was under the Touretters control – that we didn't have to do it." I told Elisabeth.

"But the context is altered." She responded, touching me back. "Here the tic has become socially appropriate. It is for the most part consensual."

Several people were exhibiting sexual touching, reaching out to breasts and genitals. Elisabeth used to work as a cocktail waitress – this was not that different.

For me the symptom built up for several hours before it erupted. At first I only needed to touch Lowell's shoulder while shouting his name, but soon it was anyone else nearby. I would reach out while talking and touch a shoulder or tap a leg if the person was sitting and people would smile and nod and touch back if they also had Tourette syndrome. Dancing was fantastic because you could make constant physical contact and feel appropriate.

While dancing with Elisabeth I leaned away to spit and she grinned at me. "I never thought I would ever say this to someone, but it's okay if you spit on me."

"But I never would," I said, shocked.

"I know that too."

Acceptance was a big theme at the conference. Sharon was like a maypole, bringing people into our group and showing them the ropes. Chris referred to her as the heart and soul of the conference. Steve talked about the "Sharon phenomena," how every male with Tourette syndrome followed her around like puppies sensing dinner.

Lowell and Laurel were making a documentary film about Tourette syndrome and Laurel's crew followed us around documenting the extraordinary communications of the Touretters.

When we all ran into each other in the hotel lobby Friday night – the adult group from the 1987 conference in Cincinnati, new friends from McLean in 1989 – there was a general group hug which lasted about twenty minutes, with people shouting at and loving each other. While we were there, several camera's followed us around panning around us, and for an ugly second we felt like specimens, not people. Jenny was outraged about the camera's and for awhile the film project was in doubt. But the emotional intensity of that moment passed and soon most of us were interacting with the camera's as being part of the experience.

Lowell had married since I had last seen him and Susanna and he were an attractive couple. "She's a demure sensitive lawyer and I'm her degenerate photojournalist husband with Tourette syndrome," Lowell explained to several people. Lowell had an article in the October 1991 issue of *In Health* about his travels with Oliver Sacks and their reunion at the conference was bittersweet. While they no longer worked together, they seemed close. But Sacks refused to participate in the film, and Lowell seemed unsure how to proceed without him.

Laurel had mild Tourette syndrome but quickly gravitated to the more severe cases. The Canadian artist Shane was like a magnet to her – drawing her into his continuously moving orbit as he Touretted around the conference, intriguing everyone who met him. Elisabeth commented to me that she had a long conversation with him one morning where he was focussed intensely on her for twenty minutes. Her hair, red it was, fascinated him and one could sense he wanted to paint her. Another woman at the conference, also intrigued by Shane, fantasized making love to him, but wondered if he could be still long enough to enjoy her. I coined the term "Charismatic Touretter" for Lowell, Shane and Sharon who seemed to attract followers wherever they went at the conference.

There was a second group of Touretters at the conference who weren't part of the adult group but observed us and joined in occasionally. One young man had severe attention deficit disorder, an associated symptom many with Tourette syndrome suffer from. He would ask you, "Where are you from?" And after you told him it would slip away from him and he would quickly ask you again, "Where are you from?" while staring at your name badge hoping to retain the information. On some level he did because he kept on coming back to the same dozen or so people trying to make contact but never quite succeeding. Another man with Tourette syndrome was abrasive and self pitying and would lie about who he knew at the conference. At one point, minutes after whining to me about his problems, he was telling my mother what good friends we had became, even though it was apparent to everyone (but him) that I detested him. At one point he said to me and several other people, "You think I'm a jerk, right?"

"No, I think you're an ass." I responded, regretting it immediately. The next morning another man told me how much the self pitier had liked my honesty and wanted to visit me. I decided not to give him my number.

There was an older population at the conference, the generation diagnosed in the 1960's, middle aged and in many cases past the worst excesses of Tourette syndrome. One man haunted me – he sat alone the entire conference, twitching by himself, and not interacting at all with anyone else. There was a dignity to him I couldn't reach, knowing that for us there would be no communication. I discussed his presence with several people, but none of us felt we could violate the wall of privacy he had built up around himself. I hope he had a good time on the edges. I felt much hope in seeing a man his age living with Tourette syndrome with his dignity intact.

Dignity. How does one live with dignity when you spit constantly, swear involuntarily, and cannot control your movements? One way was having role models with Tourette syndrome. For me, and for many my age, Orrin, a psychiatrist with severe Tourette syndrome, including coprolalia, was an inspiration. Orrin was the first person I had met with Tourette syndrome back in 1977, and his impact and advice over the years have been life affirming. Seeing Orrin with his baby Devon, his wife Jill, his fellow doctors, made one appreciate how good life could be for someone with Tourette syndrome. But I also remembered talks with Orrin when he discussed his inner demons, and I knew that there was more to the picture than what showed.

For the younger generation the role model was of course Jim Eisenreich, the baseball player who was becoming increasingly involved with the Tourette Syndrome Association. Jim's willingness to give of himself impressed me at the conference, and what I felt was almost a humility about his interactions with the more severe Touretters made me admire him but also feel great sorrow. His profession made him larger than life but he was also as needy as the rest of us and didn't have the permission to express it that the rest of us did in the group.

In any group of people with Tourette syndrome the issue of the 'super Touretter' comes up. It had a double meaning: On one hand there was the sense of it that Oliver Sacks had made of people whose rapidity and improvisations improved their lives. But there was also the people with severe Tourette syndrome who were very high functioning in an assimilated way. As an artist, a writer and a musician, I liked the concept that this deficit was also a blessing. But then I would meet someone like Kathy, whose obsessions had led to anorexia and whose daughter was developing tics and wondered how anyone in their right mind could see any beauty or good in this awful disorder.

"How can you laugh about it?" Somebody once asked me.

"Because if I don't laugh, I would cry." I replied.

In the tears was beauty too. At the previous conference I had been in the middle of my alcoholism, drinking continually from morning to night, not really able to focus in on the bigger picture. The group was self contained – we didn't share or interact much with the normals or even the Touretters who didn't 'fit in.' When shortly after the 1987 conference one of those Touretters who didn't fit in committed suicide, I entered one of my bleakest moments, reassessing my life and ultimately finding it wanting. For my life to have meaning I had to be able to share it; to communicate my experience and the experience of the people I knew with Tourette syndrome to the world at large. But the communication was a painful process, and for me, creating was an awful empty experience filled with pain and self-loathing. At the conference, whether it was because I was sober or because much of my creation was behind me (for the present) I felt a joy in each interaction realizing that this whole experience of being with people with Tourette syndrome was a gift. I could learn from them and they from me and things could be a lot better for us all.

But how to make it work - how to fit into a world which on the one hand understood Tourette syndrome more than it had and at the same time found coprolalia 'politically incorrect?' It would take a different kind of strength, a group experience rather than an individual one and the political subtext of the conference was the adult population taking charge of their own destinies.

Friday night about midnight we were in the hospitality suite with the film crew. We had requested that they put away the cameras after thirty minutes and let us be ourselves without being in the center of the goldfish bowl. Near the end Laurel dropped her bombshell. "If you could get rid of your Tourette, would you?"

There was a stunned silence in the room as we considered her question. It was an amazing one for it encompassed the totality of the Tourette experience, a disease that for better or worse had a creative aspect to it. Christian answered first that for him life was more interesting with his Tourette syndrome; that to live without it would in some way diminish his being. Kathy sat crying and after the crew left said in horror, "How could anyone ask such an awful question? Of course I would rather not have it."

There was a generational side to the question. For those of us who had lived to our late twenties and early thirties with this beast the worst was behind us, the excesses of Tourette syndrome burnt out or under control. But for those of us facing raising children, having families with the genetic scarlet letter of DNA abnormality passed onto our tender tiny loved ones, there was no way we wanted this *thing*, this disease to exist beyond us. It was a profound moment and I found myself going up to my room shortly after this conversation feeling the most awful solitude. I can never truly know anyone in my life, never communicate and the pain in that room was more than I could bear.

Sleep heals. For me, fatigue makes all of my symptoms worse, and a good nights sleep is of more benefit than any drug. I slept well and woke up less confused, less on the edge as John would say, then the night before. But I also woke knowing that this day would bring the emotional highpoint of the conference, that after a day or two of this environment, my ability to suppress was nil. There were one hundred other Touretters in the same state. What wonders would Saturday bring, and what terrors?

The banquet Saturday night was simply astonishing. Echo phenomena, commentary, involuntary heckling of the speakers, people moving about the dining hall stamping their feet, shouting, touching each other, and a sense of barely controlled hysteria. I found myself sitting next to Cynthia, who had a napkin wadded up and hanging out of her nostrils. "Are we putting things up our nose, Adam?"

"No. I'm not." I replied.

"Say yes or I have to keep on asking." Then she noticed my spitting and spat loudly onto my shoulder. Dinner was intense.

Jenny sat next to me and told me angrily that someone from the National TSA had asked her to tell people 'to behave.' "Do they really think we're doing this deliberately?"

Debra from the film crew sat down next to me with a hand held camera and asked if she could film my reactions and comments to the dinner. We sat down at a less busy table and Elisabeth joined us. "You're pretty wired?"

"I feel like I'm going to explode. I want to move and shout and I'm restraining myself."

"Why?"

"I'm not sure. A false sense of dignity to be kept?"

After dinner we were entertained by a high school choir. Greeted with a series of obscenities, shouts and hoots the choir began to sing a series of patriotic hymns. I had an incredible urge to scream at them and I headed for the exit, muttering to myself under my breath, "Burn the flag."

In the hallway Elisabeth joined me and as the choir exited the hall, I began to shake from the effort of suppressing. Elisabeth placed her hand over my mouth and I wordlessly screamed into it. I had never felt so supported in all my years with Tourette syndrome. Here was someone who knew what I was going through and accepted it. I had to run to a meeting of writers for the anthology you are now reading and managed to dance with Elisabeth in the hotel disco.

At the meeting of writers we discussed the concept of the book and passed around completed chapters. Christian was very taken with Kevin's piece and asked to take it home with him to Norway. Maura and John were very taken with Christian and the feeling of love among the people with Tourette syndrome – the Touretters as Oliver Sacks had once dubbed us, filled the room rising above to the hotel and the surrounding area. We could do anything that night. What we did was dance.

Dancing a slow dance with Elisabeth I moved away occa-

191

sionally to have full body tics, a jerking movement of my entire back. After we danced I danced with Sharon, with Shelly, with several people whose names I never got. I sat with Elisabeth and her mother Mary, and we were joined by Lowell and his wife Suzanne.

Shane darted by; Dan grabbed a crotch or two; Cynthia pulled something out her nose and I marveled aloud at the wonder of it all. These were the dearest people in my life and I had only known most of them for three days.

That night Elisabeth and I talked until dawn, and as much as I wanted to, I knew I couldn't touch her. She could touch me, hand hitting my knee to emphasize a point; but I had to behave and control my urge to throw my arms around her. I knew that if I touched her once I would have to continue and that permission hadn't been given. It was different from tic suppression - it was tic substitution as I found myself more vocal than usual, my voice modulating in new ways.

The next morning, after five hours sleep I found Elisabeth and we continued to talk, first at breakfast then at brunch. Saying goodbye to her was one of the hardest things I had ever done in my life as I felt acceptance in human form slip away.

That night Christian and Paul, from Australia, and I went to dinner. Paul was unsure about leaving the hotel grounds. "Paul's nervous," He Touretted to himself repeatedly.

"Relax. We'll go for Mexican." At the restaurant I said to the hostess, "You're in luck. All three of us have severe Tourette syndrome."

"Oh," she said grinning. "My girlfriend works at the Hilton. She said you guys are a lot of fun!"

At dinner we attempted to keep Paul from jabbing at his eyes with a fork or touching the candle with his hand. All three of us drank diet cokes and the waiter didn't seem bothered by our swearing. Christian was swearing in English and Norwegian,

Paul was muttering in Aussie slang and I tossed in my regular four letter Anglo-Saxisms. Life was grand.

Keeping in touch with people after the conference I learned that everybody had a similar experience on their way home. Stopping at a coffee shop or a gas station, there was a stunned moment when we realized that we were surrounded by people who didn't have Tourette syndrome. After the three days at the conference we had quickly adapted to a world view where Tourette syndrome was the norm. If only the rest of the world would see it that way!

My learnings from Alcoholic's Anomynous teach me to live one day at a time. My Tourette syndrome changes daily, waxing and waning with its own internal rhythms and changing to suit the stress level in my life. For today I, and those I love, live with Tourette syndrome. Tomorrow?

AFTERTHOUGHTS ON LIVING WITH TOURETTE SYNDROME

by

John S. Hilkevich
and
Adam Ward Seligman

By living with Tourette syndrome we mean not just those who have the disorder, but also their parents, spouses, siblings, teachers, counselors and any others who interact with Tourette syndrome persons. Struck by Adam De-Prince's labeling of Tourette syndrome as "unendearing," we were reminded how, indeed, we can be very difficult and an outright pain to live with. Even more troublesome to

195

others is that the mirroring aspect of Tourette syndrome, the mimicking of sounds, words, and behavior, are not just confined to the world of sight, sound, touch and movement but rattles the psyche as well. We learned to take personal inventory when we are bothered by another's defects of character, realizing that much of what we see in others is a reflection of our own issues.

A friend of ours, whose Tourette syndrome noises are loud enough that we can tell if he is home before approaching his front door, told us of how a blind man had stopped him to ask if he had Tourette syndrome. When our friend answered yes, the man replied, "I have heard about Tourette syndrome. You must have a difficult time." This ironic remark by an endearing blind man about an unendearing disease testifies to his keen vision. Our friend and this man were seeing reflections of each other's lives.

There is little endearment triggered by a seven year old who, after biting away his nails, could not stop chewing the skin off the sides of his fingers. Or by a newly married woman whose husband left her because of her violent temper and three hour long daily walks to which he was not invited. Or a young child who must keep tapping his feet in quiet places and has not worn socks in months because he "can't stand them." Or the adult who compulsively spits into his dinner plate while eating. Instead there is confusion, resentment, ridicule. How does one live with this disorder?

In late 1989 when I first went public with my Tourette syndrome story, I received an explosion of letters of support from the Tourette syndrome community. Many offered advice, some useful and some for which I was not yet ready. One wrote, "I tried suppression for many years but I couldn't stand the pain of holding back the explosion within me. So after many years I followed a different road. As I 'let go' I was stared at more often but I also began overtly talking to others about Tourette syndrome as well. This approach had an unexpected, positive reaction for me because I went from hiding and being ashamed to literally coming out and educating people and being unafraid. Letting my tics out does keep me in balance. As much as we wish to explain Tourette syndrome and what goes on inside us to one who doesn't have it, they can never really comprehend the feelings. I too could not differentiate between what was me and what was Tourette syndrome, so I couldn't really worry about someone else's understanding what I myself didn't fully comprehend. Meanwhile, try not to take Tourette syndrome too seriously. If you do – it will consume you." (Quoted from Bob Nast with permission.)

Tourette syndrome people know how to lighten up about their disorder as you can garner from reading the chapter, *In the Group*. Part of the healing process of pain involves putting a different frame around it, giving it different meaning and putting it to productive use. The reader can see how the contributors to this book have done just that in their own unique ways.

The Second International Scientific Symposium on Tourette Syndrome was held in 1991. It helped define the direction of Tourette syndrome research for this decade. Genetic and pharmacologic treatment strategies will continue to be developed and remain an essential path to help afflicted persons live with Tourette syndrome. But there are "back-door" ways to changing neurological symptoms that side step the direct hammer of neuroleptic medications, such as nutrition, exercise, allergen avoidance, recreational pursuits and others which increase brain serotonin (a neurotransmitter that enhances behavioral control) and these also should be given proportionate attention in this proclaimed "Decade of the Brain."

The symposium reiterated the many studies documenting the high correlations between Tourette syndrome, obsessive-compulsive disorder, attention deficit disorder, hyperactivity, learning disability, anxiety, depression and other disorders. As Tourette syndrome and associated disorders gain recognition as one of the most prevalent genetic aberrations, our nation's schools must wake up and look at the one percent or more of its children who are affected by some Tourette syndrome related symptoms and see as well as our friend's blind man.

Using the term addiction in a broad, nonclinical sense, and recognizing the differences between addiction, compulsions, obsessions and tics, there is an addictive flavor to Tourette syndrome. Addictions to gambling, eating, sex, risk-taking, and other activities as well as to chemicals are possible because these change our neurochemistry and what we really become addicted to are these changes. Thus it is no accident that some Tourette syndrome persons follow one of the many "12 Step Programs" in the form of Overeaters Anonymous, Gamblers Anonymous, or Alcoholics Anonymous. Many have expressed curiosity in our applying the 12 Steps to Tourette syndrome itself, which resulted from our years of fighting it and finally realizing that we, by ourselves, were indeed powerless over the Tourette syndrome in us. A surrendering of that and all of our lives to our Higher Power and the concomitant self-inventorying, connecting with others, and getting the message out, actualized a liberation of our social, emotional, mental and spiritual selves. This book was part of that "stepping out" for us.

The medical and mental health communities are venturing to make sense of Tourette syndrome. For those of us afflicted with it and those who live and work with us, making sense of it may be less important than finding ways to use it, even to be empowered by it. That is what kept Frankl and thousands of others alive in the Nazi concentration camps where it was much easier to let go and die. We can integrate and even be grateful for suffering and pain that makes our lives better than it would have been without the trials and tribulations.

Joseph Campbell wrote of the hero's quest, his journey to find meaning, and through it, rebirth. All of our writers are taking their own version of that quest and with its many different manifestations, it occurs to us that Tourette syndrome is the disorder with a thousand faces. We spoke one night before the fireplace and discussed the differences between our western culture, which fears those who are different, and shamanistic cultures which often take those who are afflicted with neurological impairments and turn them into medicine people. The shaman with seizures, the medicine man who twitches violently, the religious leader who stutters when excited, are thus fully integrated into the life of the community. John's search for spiritual meaning, or Adam's quest for an environment in which he felt safe to live his life, reflect this tendency of those with Tourette syndrome to find a niche in our increasingly diverse society.

The word "Touretter" is used by several of our writers. Others prefer "persons with Tourette syndrome." There is room for both points of view in this book because as victims of intolerance it is important for us to accept others with the generosity they often deny us. We are struck by Wayne Martin's use of the term Tourette American – recognizing that we are truly cultural and political entities not just people who happen to move to a different drummer. At the same time whether we are Touretters or people with Tourette syndrome, we are also just plain folks trying to live a normal life. As we try to imitate those monkeys and speak no evil think no evil hear no evil, we become just like all our non -Tourette brothers and sisters who hopefully can learn from us as we learn from them.

As an afterthought, that is a message to our readers who may not know anyone with Tourette syndrome and wonder why they should read this book. After all, we all have our burdens that need healing. We all have monkeys we are trying not to think about.

But when we cannot not think of them, we can take a break to watch them. Sometimes monkeys do some pretty funny things and make us smile.

Hope Press Books

"A masterwork"

J. Lejune
Archives of Genetique

"Best Health Book of the Year"

American Book Dealers Exchange

"Thank you for writing this book. For the first time in my life I finally really understand my child and my family."

Parent of a Tourette syndrome child

RYAN - A Mother's Story of Her Hyperactive/Tourette Syndrome Child
by *Susan Hughes*

"This is a book that I can't wait for my family and friends to read. It gives insight, support, understanding and pertinent information in a positive, caring and determined manner. I would have all the educators read it! It would be a great resource in child development classes. I can't get the book out of my mind. It brings to the surface all the feelings, emotions and frustrations that I and my family live with every day."

Mother of a Tourette syndrome child

"Mothers can be a great source of wisdom. Doctors may listen but they do not always hear what mothers are saying. The story Susan Hughes tells is typical of what thousands of mothers of hyperactive or Tourette syndrome children have endured..."

David E. Comings, M.D.

"The language is clear, and medical and psychiatric terms are well defined. The tone is positive and supportive toward the audience of mothers and their troubled children. However, the author does not sugarcoat realistic problems but acknowledges the numerous difficulties in rearing such children and offers practical suggestions..."

Sherry. L. Taggard, M.D.
Journal of Clinical Psychiatry

HI, I'M ADAM - A Child's Story of Tourette Syndrome
by *Adam Buehrens*

ADAM AND THE MAGIC MARBLE
A Magical Adventure
by *Adam and Carol Buehrens*

"Adam - I really thank you for writing this book because I know it will help children who have Tourette syndrome to better understand themselves. It will also help their parents, teachers and friends to understand how

203

they feel about Tourettes. I hope every newly diagnosed person with Tourette will get a copy of this book and read it"

Harvey Dean
President, Tourette Syndrome Association

Hi, I'm Adam - "Read this to your child... Have your child read it to you... but however you read it, READ IT and grow in the knowledge that these unique children are just like all the other children on this earth – special and deserve our support, love, and understanding."

Adam and the Magic Marble - "This is a MUST book for anyone, adult or child, who has a disability, knows someone who has a disability, or can read!"

Catherine Woktkun MA,Ed.
A Parents Guide to *Kids n Stuff*

ECHOLALIA by *Adam Ward Seligman*

"Knowing about Tourette syndrome did not prepare me for what I found in ECHOLALIA: The outward signs of Tourette are hard to miss, but the internal symptoms, the continual mental disquiet, are unguessable. I've watched as Adam Seligman's spirit has bested Tourette and now, I marvel as his talent inspires and educates. ECHOLALIA is a disturbing, heartening and not-to-be-missed experience."

Ed Asner

"This debut novel, by Adam Ward Seligman, provides a fascinating glimpse into the world of Tourette syndrome and its impact on the creative process. The slant on the subject is fresh, the writing style engaging, and the insights rare and disturbing. I look forward to hearing more from this talented writer."

Sue Grafton
Author of *'H' is for Homicide*

"ECHOLALIA has made visible something most people don't know about and you've done it in a personal yet general way, with a fine sense of pacing and poetic grace."

William Wharton
Author of *Birdy, Dad* and *In a Midnight Clear*

"Adam Seligman's novel ECHOLALIA is a first novel in more than one sense. It's Mr. Seligman's initial foray into publishing but, more importantly, it's one of a small group of pioneering novels that exhibit for the first time in literary history the experience of disability from an insiders point of view. Mr. Seligman combines a fascinating portrait of a character who has Tourette syndrome with a satirical look at modern day publishing where deals with Stephen Spielberg count more than the written word. Jackson Evans, saddled with worldly savoir-faire and an unseemly amount of sexual naivete in danger of derailment into perversion, struggles to accept fame, his newly diagnosed condition, and eventually, himself."

Victoria Ann-Lewis
Artist in Residence
Marc Taper Forum

"Jazz lurks in the background of ECHOLALIA. This novel by occasional JAZZIZ contributor Adam Ward Seligman is often fascinating. Seligman, who has had the neurological disorder, Tourette syndrome, since he was a child, has written a story dealing with a fictional writer-drummer with the disease and his battle to live with himself that really lets one into the mind of a victim. This intriguing story is both entertaining and educational."

Scott Yanow
JAZZIZ Magazine

"This aggressive, engaging and hugely ambitious novel about a best-selling author with Tourette syndrome almost accomplishes the impossible...writer Adam Ward Seligman transforms this complex brain disorder into a vision of the world that bears as much relevance to readers without Tourette syndrome as to those who have it. This literary leap, in which Seligman explains the realities of Tourette and fictionalizes its deeper meanings, is the rare gift he brings to the novel form...This is a rare, challenging work by a talented writer with exceptional vision."

Patricia Holt
San Francisco Chronicle

NOTES

NOTES

NOTES

NOTES

Order Form

Tourette Syndrome and Human Behavior
David E. Comings, M.D.
1S softback $39.95
ISBN 1-878267-27-2
#_____ $_____

Search for the Tourette Syndrome and Human Behavior Genes
David E. Comings, M.D.
8S softback $29.95
ISBN 1-878267-41-8
#_____ $_____
8H hardback $34.00
ISBN 1-878267-36-1
#_____ $_____

The Gene Bomb
David E. Comings, M.D.
9S softback $25.00
ISBN 1-878267-39-6
#_____ $_____
9H hardback $29.95
ISBN 1-878267-38-8
#_____ $_____

RYAN — A Mother's Story of Her Hyperactive-Tourette Syndrome Child
Susan Hughes
2S softback $9.95
ISBN 1-878267-26-4
#_____ $_____

What Makes Ryan Tick? A Family's Triumph over TS and ADHD
Susan Hughes
10S softback $14.95
ISBN 1-878267-35-3
#_____ $_____

Teaching the Tiger - A Handbook for Individuals Involved in the Education of Students with Attention Deficit Disorder, Tourette Syndrome or Obsessive-Compulsive Disorder
Marilyn P. Dornbush, Ph.D
Sheryl K. Pruitt, M.Ed.
7S softback $35.00
ISBN 1-878267-34-5
#_____ $_____

Don't Think About Monkeys - Extraordinary Stories by People with Tourette Syndrome
Adam Ward Seligman
John S. Hiolkevich
6S softback $12.95
ISBN 1-878267-33-7
#_____ $_____

A.D.D. Kaleidoscope - The Many Facets of Adult AttentionDeficit Disorder
Joan Andrews, M.S., MFCC
Denis E. Davis, M.S. MFCC
19S softbka $24.95
ISBN 18782267-035
#_____ $_____

Check-up from the Neck-up Ensuring Mental Health in the Next Millennium
Joan Andrews, M.S., MFCC
Denis E. Davis, M.S. MFCC
15S Softback $19.95
ISBN 1-878267-09-4
#_____ $_____

ADHD A Survival Guide for Parents and Teachers
Richard Lougy, MFT
David Rosenthal, M.D.
18S softback $24.95
ISBN 1-878267-43-4
#_____ $_____

Overload Attention Deficit Disorder and the Adictive Brain David Miller
Kenneth Blum, Ph.D.
17S softback $24.95
ISBN 18782267-426
#_____ $_____

Dysinhibition Syndrome - How to Handle Anger and Rage in Your Child or Spouse
Rose Wood
12S softback $24.95
ISBN 1-878267-08-6
#_____ $_____

Hi, I'm Adam - A Child's Book about Tourette Syndrome Adam Buehrens
4S softback $4.95
ISBN 1-878267-29-9
#_____ $_____

Adam and the Magic Marble
Adam Buehrens
Carol Buehrens
4B softback $6.95
ISBN 1-878267-30-2
#_____ $_____

Subtotal for Books _____

th Class: $4.00 1st item $1.00 each additional item
. Ground: $6.00 1st item $1.00 each additional item
. Air: $10.00 1st item $2.00 each additional item

California residents add 8.25% sales tax _____

Total _____

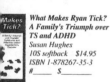

_____ City: _____

ss: _____ State: _____ Zip: _____

ry (other than U.S.A.): _____ Check Enclosed _____ **or**

_____ Expiration Date _____ Visa ___ MC ___

d to: ☐┬○ **Hope Press** P.O.Box 188, Duarte, CA 91009-0188

Fill out this form with credit card # and FAX it to 626-358-3520
order on the web at **http://www.hopepress.com**

ent Books is our Canadian distributor 1-800-209-9182 FAX 416-537-9499

Order Form

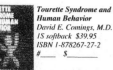

Tourette Syndrome and Human Behavior
David E. Comings, M.D.
1S softback $39.95
ISBN 1-878267-27-2
#____ $_____

Search for the Tourette Syndrome and Human Behavior Genes
David E. Comings, M.D.
8S softback $29.95
ISBN 1-878267-41-8
#____ $_____
8H hardback $34.00
ISBN 1-878267-36-1
#____ $_____

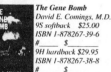

The Gene Bomb
David E. Comings, M.D.
9S softback $25.00
ISBN 1-878267-39-6
#____ $_____
9H hardback $29.95
ISBN 1-878267-38-8
#____ $_____

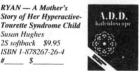

RYAN — A Mother's Story of Her Hyperactive-Tourette Syndrome Child
Susan Hughes
2S softback $9.95
ISBN 1-878267-26-4
#____ $_____

What Makes Ryan Tick? A Family's Triumph over TS and ADHD
Susan Hughes
10S softback $14.95
ISBN 1-878267-35-3
#____ $_____

Teaching the Tiger - A Handbook for Individuals Involved in the Education of Students with Attention Deficit Disorder, Tourette Syndrome or Obsessive-Compulsive Disorder
Marilyn P. Dornbush, Ph.D
Sheryl K. Pruitt, M.Ed.
7S softback $35.00
ISBN 1-878267-34-5
#____ $_____

Don't Think About Monkeys - Extraordinary Stories by People with Tourette Syndrome
Adam Ward Seligman
John S. Hiolkevich
6S softback $12.95
ISBN 1-878267-33-7
#____ $_____

A.D.D. Kaleidoscope - The Many Facets of Adult AttentionDeficit Disorder
Joan Andrews, M.S., MFCC
Denis E. Davis, M.S. MFCC
19S softback $24.95
ISBN 18782267-035
#____ $_____

Check-up from the Neck-up Ensuring Mental Health in the Next Millennium
Joan Andrews, M.S., MFCC
Denis E. Davis, M.S. MFCC
15S Softback $19.95
ISBN 1-878267-09-4
#____ $_____

ADHD A Survival Guide for Parents and Teachers
Richard Lougy, MFT
David Rosenthal, M.D.
18S softback $24.95
ISBN 1-878267-43-4
#____ $_____

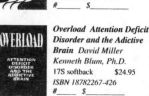

Overload Attention Deficit Disorder and the Adictive Brain David Miller
Kenneth Blum, Ph.D.
17S softback $24.95
ISBN 18782267-426
#____ $_____

Dysinhibition Syndrome - How to Handle Anger and Rage in Your Child or Spouse
Rose Wood
12S softback $24.95
ISBN 1-878267-08-6
#____ $_____

Hi, I'm Adam - A Child's Book about Tourette Syndrome Adam Buehrens
4S softback $4.95
ISBN 1-878267-29-9
#____ $_____

Adam and the Magic Marble
Adam Buehrens
Carol Buehrens
4B softback $6.95
ISBN 1-878267-30-2
#____ $_____

Subtotal for Books _____

ourth Class: $4.00 lst item $1.00 each additional item
P.S. Ground: $6.00 lst item $1.00 each additional item
P.S. Air: $10.00 lst item $2.00 each additional item _____

California residents
add 8.25% sales tax _____

Total _____

ne:_____

City: _____

ress:_____

State:_____ Zip: _____

ntry (other than U.S.A.): _____

Check Enclosed _____ **or**

#_____ Expiration Date _____ Visa ___ MC ___

send to: ☐─○ **Hope Press** P.O.Box 188, Duarte, CA 91009-0188

or   Fill out this form with credit card # and FAX it to **626-358-3520**

or   order on the web at **http://www.hopepress.com**

Parent Books is our Canadian distributor 1-800-209-9182 FAX 416-537-9499